D0467706

For my (lean) and loving father. I am in awe of you and the lives you've saved, always with such baffling humility. I am so proud to be the daughter of such a pioneering surgeon. Thank you for embracing me just as I am, warts and all. Daddy – you are my first and greatest love.

The Louise Parker Method

LEAN
for
LIFE

Transform your
body in 6 weeks

Protect the
results forever

MITCHELL BEAZLEY

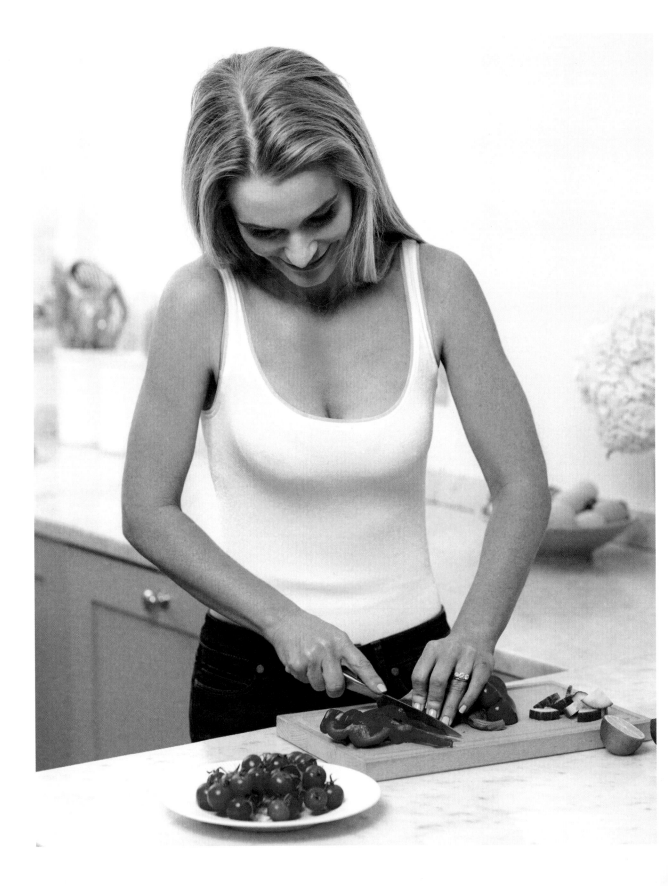

CONTENTS

HOW TO USE THIS BOOK

The Louise Parker Method has transformed thousands of bodies and lifestyles just like yours over the last 20 years. I'm delighted to be sharing my Method with you in this book, taking you directly to a body that thrills you as a new way of living simultaneously falls into place.

You'll discover beautiful meals that you love and workouts that make you feel alive. You'll learn that weight loss should be nurturing, not punishing. Once you've reached your most aspirational body, I'll show you how to create the lifestyle to sustain it. This blueprint for lasting success is what sets the method apart and why thousands of our clients have raved that 'I just wished I'd known 10 years ago how simple it can be'. It's a lot simpler to be 'Lean for Life' than you'd ever imagine.

There are four building block chapters for the pillars of my method: Live Well, Think Successfully, Eat Beautifully and Work Out Intelligently. Each pillar seamlessly links together to make the journey to your ultimate potential achievable, practicable and thrilling.

With the knowledge in place, the last section of the book focuses on the programme itself, a Transform phase lasting 42 days. Finally, the Louise Parker Lifestyle will help you to adopt these new habits forever.

IN THE TRANSFORM PHASE, YOU'LL SIMPLY:

THINK SUCCESSFULLY	LIVE WELL	EAT BEAUTIFULLY	WORK OUT INTELLIGENTLY
★ Adopt a positive mindset and assume success	★ Declutter your surroundings	★ Eat 3 meals and 2 snacks per day. You have a choice of 80 recipes, each super simple and quick to prepare	★ Weave activity into your everyday, with an absolute minimum of 10,000 steps per day. Aim as high as you can
★ Make time for simple pleasures every single day	★ Digital detox after 9pm every night		
★ Deal with and dissolve all your worries	★ Sleep 7 hours a night	★ Start your day with 'Lemonize' and stay well hydrated throughout	★ Complete a minimum of 15 minutes of my Louise Parker Method home workouts
★ Keep positive, inspiring company	★ Take a 'brain-nap' for 20 minutes a day		
1	**2**	**3**	**4**

INTRODUCTION

I feel happiest when I'm light on my toes, bursting with energy, lean and toned. It's when I'm living my best life, in a positive state of mind and achieving my full potential. And feeling my absolute best cannot come at the price of obsessing over my diet and exercise. To be fit, happy and free, I need freedom from the tedious cycle of dieting. That's why I devised the Louise Parker Method.

My Method is about more than just losing weight. It's about living a lifestyle that sustains you in optimum health, peak performance and clarity of mind so you are absolutely brimming with vitality. The side-effect of this lifestyle is that your body will transform into one that is exceptionally lean, sculpted, strong and graceful. And because you've changed the habits of your lifestyle, the results stick.

The results truly do last – because for once you're not relying on willpower to succeed and you're permanently changing your habits. You're going to need to put in a little effort up front as you get going, and then the habits take over and look after you forever. Motivation is temporary; habits sustain your results for all time.

I no longer worry about my weight, what I'm eating or what I should or shouldn't be doing. The healthy habits are just that – habits that would now be impossible to break. I enjoy a normal life, with croissants on Sundays and rosé on Fridays. I don't drink kale juice, eat my meals from Tupperware or train for two hours a day. No food I adore is off-limits and I never feel guilty about what I eat. I'm happy in my skin, wear what I want to wear and don't dread the bikini season as I did two decades ago.

Thousands of my clients have achieved this too – and there's absolutely no reason why you won't be next. The success rate of the Louise Parker Method is extraordinary, both in terms of jaw-dropping results and the longevity of them. After all, it's all about ending dieting for good.

I spent so many years held back by the distraction of dieting and the pursuit of a body that for some reason I couldn't attain. The roller coaster of deprivation and indulgence left me floored with tiredness and depressed. It's amazing how you can tread water through life because you've neither the energy nor the confidence for it.

I only wish I'd known then what I know now: that gaining and keeping a fabulous body needn't be agony – it's not meant to be hard. And that if it's hard, you won't sustain it; and if you can't sustain it, you're back to square one. I'd have told myself to go and get the body I want, once and for all, in the most sensible way there is. Don't stop until you have it, and practise being consistent. Take the most direct route. Create habits that you love, and that work for you. I'd have told myself to do it with food that I actually enjoy eating, and to focus on creating the habits of eating well. I'd have said stop the intermittent gruelling workouts and just do a little something every day. I'd have spoken to myself more kindly, as I would to a daughter or a friend.

I have a very busy life, and no more time to focus on my body than you do. Everything I put in has to give me three times that amount back, in energy and output. I know I create more time for myself by living this lifestyle. I don't spend a minute longer in the kitchen or working out than I have to and, because the Method truly fits in around my life, it's just what I do now.

I have three wonderful daughters, a husband I adore, a company that's thriving, a team of 50 amazing colleagues and a gaggle of gorgeous girlfriends. I'm extraordinarily lucky, although I've a lot on my plate. I've definitely strived for every serving and I don't want to lean back from the table. I'm a modern mum, I guess, and I want it all. It's imperative that I feel fabulous and energetic, to keep up with all I have going on.

Motivation is temporary; habits sustain your results for all time

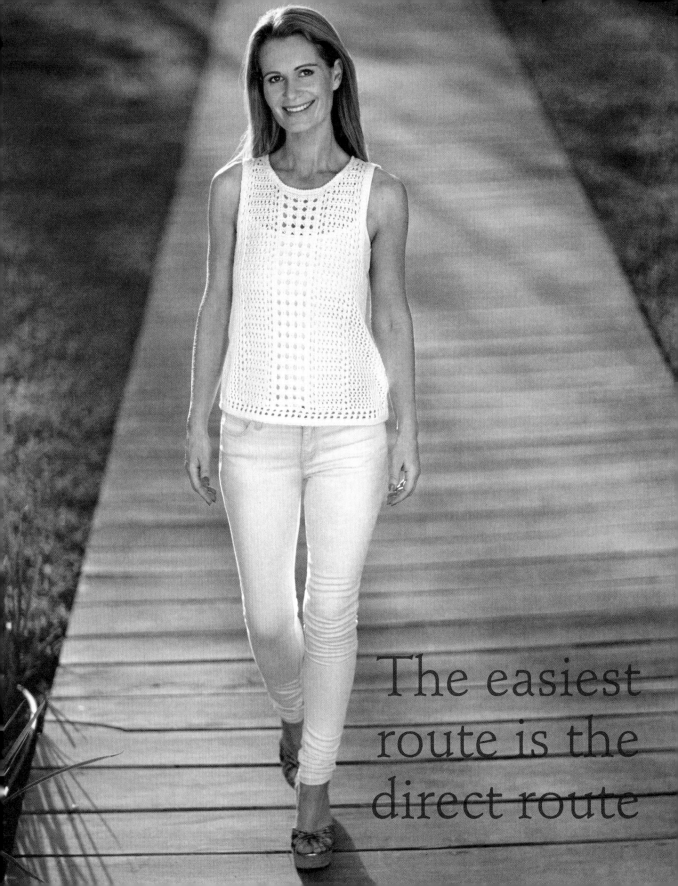

The easiest
route is the
direct route

When I've a spring in my step, I lean into everything and I'm just better at life – I'm a more loving wife, a more patient mother, a more inspiring boss, a lovelier sister, daughter and friend. I actually need to operate in this zone where I feel amazing on most days. There's no way I can keep up with the pace of my life if I'm not firing on all cylinders.

I'm not an ex-dancer or athlete, and I've never worked at a gym. At school I was kissing boys, smoking behind the bike sheds and bunking off PE. My voyage into fitness came about simply because I wanted to lose weight. In the final year of my drama degree at the University of London I decided to start working out because I loathed being plump and lacked confidence on the stage. I'd started my first diet at 14 at boarding school, and with each one I'd gained a couple of pounds. I was never fat, but I hated being curvy – as you do at 21. Looking back now, I realize I looked lovely.

I became fascinated by how just a few weeks of exercise classes manipulated my body, and the effect this had on my confidence. Within weeks I'd enrolled on a personal training course, primarily to pay off my student loan. It was such an unusual course to study in London 20 years ago and, with so few personal trainers around, it was more or less exclusively a service for the rich and famous. My clients were glamorous, challenging and very demanding. I was captivated and fascinated in equal measure, and my appetite to develop the most effective system grew every year. I think being a normal girl, and not a gym-bunny, enabled me to really understand my clients. They wanted what I wanted – to spend no more effort than was necessary to get a fabulous result.

The years flew by and I soon forgot about acting – I'd found my calling. I developed my signature programme, 'The Intensive', 15 years ago and set up my company when I could no longer keep up with the waiting list. I now run the company with my husband Paul, who left his City job four years ago to help us keep up with the ever-increasing demand for our Method. To date, over 11,000 people in more than 48 countries have completed a Louise Parker programme.

I've spent 20 years learning, researching, testing and improving my system, and everything I have learned has become the Louise Parker Method. I'm so proud of the thousands of lives we've already changed, and believe that this book will help many thousands more to lose body fat, attain a body they are just thrilled with and create healthy lifestyle habits that last.

THE PROMISE

The Louise Parker Method is a style of living that transports you to the best of health, body and mindset in the quickest, safest and most intelligent way possible. Once you reach your absolute potential, it will support you there for the rest of your life.

Your body will radically transform into one that is super-lean, strong and lithe. I will sculpt you into the most graceful version of yourself, whatever your age or starting point. My Method is powerful and won't be held back by anything that you perceive as an obstacle – your age, your genes, your metabolism, your injury, your demanding lifestyle.

I will teach you the most effective way to achieve results that you never thought possible, in the most time-efficient manner. I passionately believe that there is no faster way to achieve such an impressive transformation of your body in a style that wisely protects your health, metabolism and happiness whilst dramatically improving your health.

The Louise Parker Method will smartly guide you through the four pillars of its success – each one connecting and seamlessly linking together to make your journey to your ultimate potential a do-able, practicable and thrilling one. You'll discover healthy meals that you love and workouts that make you feel alive. You'll learn that weight loss should be nurturing, not punishing.

Once you've reached your most aspirational body, I'll teach you how to sustain it with as little effort as possible. You'll be living a lifestyle that's totally normal (not a chia seed in sight), whilst wearing your skinny jeans and enjoying celebrations, absolutely guilt-free. When my Method becomes part of you, you'll wish you'd discovered it years ago.

WHAT IS THE LOUISE PARKER METHOD?

There are two phases to the Louise Parker Method:

TRANSFORM   Taking the direct route to your best body

LIFESTYLE   Protecting your results for life

My Method is a style of living that perfectly blends eating beautifully, working out intelligently and embracing a positive mindset and lifestyle. It's the powerful balance of these four pillars that make it a recipe for success.

Everything you learn in the Transform Phase will form the foundation of your New Normal. Whilst you're sculpting your body, you're simultaneously creating habits that will last a lifetime. The beautiful meals and the habit of exercise will now be part of your life and simply what you do. You'll continue with a positive mindset and lifestyle habits, and will really take pleasure in looking after yourself.

The Lifestyle Plan is about freedom from trend dieting, where you'll learn the art of maintaining a lean body in the most intelligent and effortless way – it's about living your best life as the most brilliant version of yourself and relaxing into it.

Finally I will teach you true balance. Gone are the days when you let rip for weeks and vow to go on a restrictive regime every Monday. It doesn't work, it's punishing and utterly boring and you deserve something so much better.

It's the precision of each ingredient that gives my Method the power to transform you, swiftly and simply. I'll help you with all four pillars of the Louise Parker Method by teaching you why each one is essential for success. I'll then show you how to put each habit into practice in the easiest way possible, for the rest of your life.

It's about living your best life as the most brilliant version of yourself

THE FOUR PILLARS

1 THINK SUCCESSFULLY

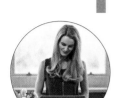

In order to achieve something that you've never achieved before, you're going to have to think in a way that you've never thought before. You're going to take a giant leap of faith and assume nothing but success. Your body will follow what your mind tells it to, so if you keep telling yourself that you will succeed and change for good, then you will.

Success is a decision, and we're going to make success inevitable. You will have a clear vision of what you want to achieve – one that's in such sharp focus that you can see every detail and almost feel it in your bones. As you continue to visualize it, you'll take a step closer to it every day.

2 LIVE WELL

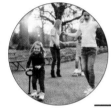

You'll create lifestyle habits that last. They have a scientific and a feel-good purpose, and they're the glue that makes the other pillars stand the test of time. So you'll create them in the Transform Phase and then, as you ease into the Lifestyle Plan, you'll need to tend to them, too – always nurturing them so that your life and body continue to evolve.

Managing stress and sleeping well affect the hormones that support weight loss, so it's essential that you get these under control. You'll replace clutter, chaos and disorganization with a lifestyle that is prepared, ordered and serene. Your result goes so much further than the mere aesthetic – it's a life that feels so beautiful you'll never want to go back.

3 EAT BEAUTIFULLY

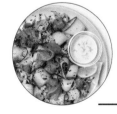

You're going to learn a simple, time-effective, beautiful style of eating lean. It's not a diet, it's just how you're going to eat from here on. You'll follow it 100 per cent of the time until your transformation is complete, and then follow it 80 per cent of the time to maintain your result. Throughout the Transform Phase you're putting into place the eating habits that will last a lifetime.

You'll love the food that you eat and you'll want to eat it forever. Each meal and snack will be beautiful and later you're going to celebrate all the good foods that are 'worth it'. I've packed as much nutrition as I can into your meals: you're going to be flooded with goodness. Each meal is precisely timed balanced with protein, carbs and fats – all in the perfect quantities to keep you in the optimal fat-burning zone. I've taken care of the science and made it as simple and normal as possible for you to follow for life.

4 WORK OUT INTELLIGENTLY

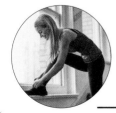

Very simply, you'll move more. You will become an active person who exercises every day. You'll slot this in as time-efficiently as possible, without having to rely on a gym.

You are going to learn concise workouts that can be done in the comfort of your own home. My Method is about getting you the most superb body and sustaining it with as little time and effort as possible. Your workouts will consist of cardio-sculpting, so whilst you're raising your heart rate and burning fat, you're also going to be honing and toning yourself to perfection.

Some days will be lighter, others more challenging, and you'll fit it around your mood and what's going on. You'll become your own personal trainer and will hold yourself accountable for what you do.

THE SCIENCE

My Method is going to beautifully weave together all the science and tricks of the trade to give you the simplest, swiftest body-transformation method there is.

What you eat is going to power your transformation. We're going to create a calorific deficit, to turn your fat-burning tap on and keep it on, until you reach your goal. The style in which you eat and the science behind the combinations and portions are going to put your body in a state where your appetite will be beautifully managed, so that you don't rely on willpower, and your hormones (ghrelin and leptin in particular – the hunger and satiety hormones respectively, see page 38) will behave and make this the most effective route to permanent weight loss.

You'll adopt a mindset that breeds success, and that keeps you powering through your programme and changes the way you think for life. You'll build habits, sleep better to regulate your hunger hormones, and manage stress to control your adrenalin and cortisol.

There's clever science behind my daily workouts that will shed your body fat and tone you within an inch of your life. We're going to optimize your afterburn and boost your metabolism, then keep it up for ever. And you won't believe how simple it is.

THE RESULTS

The results you get from following the Louise Parker Method will truly astound you. You'll be surprised at how easily they come and how do-able it all feels – you'll probably worry that it feels *too* easy.

Expect to drop one-and-a-half dress sizes in each six-week round, and be pleasantly surprised when you drop two. If you've got multiple dress sizes to drop, just keep repeating the Transform Phase until you reach your goal. If you stick to the plan, your weight loss won't slow down (this applies to 'diets' where most of the initial 'weight loss' isn't actually fat, but water and muscle).

Don't take days 'off' in between rounds, because the most direct route is the easiest route and we're stopping all this 'on' and 'off' habit for good. Try not to think of it in six-week chunks at all; focus on one day at a time. Once the train is running at high speed, keep it running. Once you stop, it wastes energy getting started again. Given that you've only got to do this once, why not just keep going and get an eye-watering, thrilling result. You really do deserve it, and it's yours for the taking if you're ready to commit.

I promise you that maintaining a size-8 body is no harder than maintaining a size-14 body – maintenance is maintenance, and when you move into the Lifestyle Plan and you're perfectly sustaining your result, it'll be no harder if you are two dress sizes smaller. People often share with me: 'I'd love to be a size ten, but I know it's

unrealistic – it'll be too hard to maintain.' Please realize that it truly isn't any harder when you're a smaller version of yourself. So if you want it, go and get it – simply stay on the train for a few more stops. Remember: it's a one-time effort and worth doing for a few more weeks, given that the results will last a lifetime.

I've never met a client who has stood in a body they've only dreamed about and has complained that it took four weeks longer than they'd hoped. We're creating a body that you're going to live in and sustain for the rest of your life, so practise consistency to get a result that properly thrills you.

If you've less weight to lose – such as 5.5kg (12lb) or under – you'll lose this on one six-week round. Don't forget that it's equally about sculpting, and you'll be rewarded with a firm, tight body. If you've 14kg (30lb) to drop, it may take one-and-a-half rounds. Four dress sizes will take two or three rounds. You get the idea. Just keep following the Method to the most consistent level you can, until you reach your target. Start once and don't stop.

Whilst most clients come to us with body transformation and fat loss as the main objectives, they leave with a long list of other benefits. I know it's tempting to focus on the fat loss, but try not to. When you change your lifestyle, the results will come your way, whether you obsess about it or not.

HERE'S WHAT TO EXPECT:

★ **Your body fat levels will plummet** as fast as physically possible, whilst protecting precious muscle mass. You'll typically lose one-and-a-half to two dress sizes on each six-week round.

★ **Your body will tighten** to a physique that is compact, strong and firm.

★ **Your visceral-fat rating will drop** (this is the hidden belly fat that surrounds your internal organs) to a healthy level, reducing the risk of heart disease, cancer, Type II diabetes, arthritis and strokes.

★ **Your energy and concentration will soar** and you'll get more done in less time.

★ **You'll boost your metabolism** (basal metabolic rate or BMR) through a stronger body.

★ **Happiness will replace moodiness** as you will no longer suffer from blood-sugar highs and lows. Your hormones will stabilize beautifully, leaving you feeling calm, yet energized and happy.

★ **Your stress levels will nosedive** as you take more time to look after yourself, eat well, exercise intelligently and get more sleep. Life will fall into perspective.

★ **Your skin will dramatically improve** as your body is flooded with vitamins, antioxidants and fluids, leaving your skin hydrated, glowing and looking many years younger.

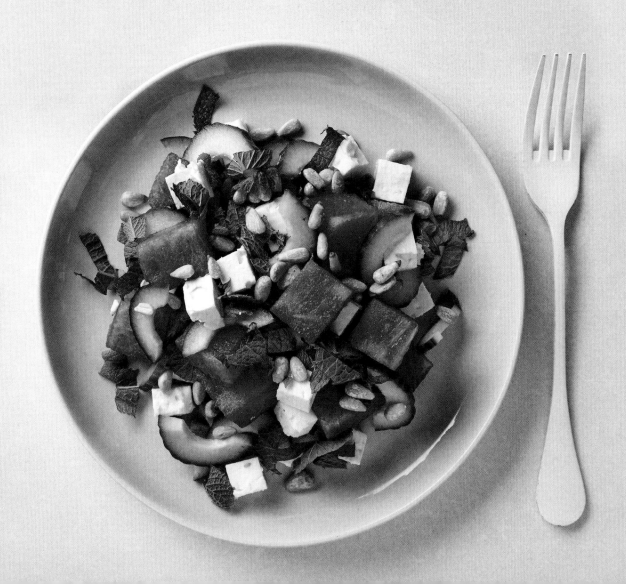

★ **Your stomach will flatten** as you radically improve your digestion and burn through abdominal fat.

★ **Cellulite will decrease** as many contributory factors are eliminated – poor diet, fad dieting, bad circulation and dehydration.

★ **Your blood will carry oxygen and nutrients** to every cell of your body, with increased blood flow and a nutrient-dense diet. Each workout will help flush cellular debris from your system.

★ **Your bone density will improve** as you increase the amount of muscle mass on your frame, reducing your risk of osteoporosis in later life.

★ **You'll feel well rested and beat exhaustion** as the quality and quantity of your sleep increase through regular exercise and improved lifestyle.

★ **You will create positive habits**, take great pride in your appearance and live in a body that feels fit, strong and beautiful.

★ **Motivation to tackle other areas of your life will kick in** as you feel empowered and in optimum health.

★ **Your sex drive will wake up and party** as your energy and confidence levels soar and your pelvic floor tightens (be warned: many clients fall pregnant towards the end of our programmes).

★ **Regular exercise will lower your resting blood pressure**, reducing your risk of cardiovascular disease and strokes. (I know, it sounds dull in comparison to the previous point.)

★ **Your lifespan and quality of life will increase** as your risk of heart disease, cancer and diabetes decreases, because you will adopt a diet rich in phytonutrients, antioxidants and vitamins, dramatically reduce your alcohol and sugar consumption and become active.

★ **You'll feel proud of setting a good example** to your family by taking great care of your body and health in a way that is fad-free, sustainable and sensible.

★ **You'll be free from the chains of trend dieting** and happy that you've found a permanent way of life that is practical, sustainable and satisfying.

This list of promises is literally life-changing and, for you to own it, I'll need your undivided attention throughout your Transform Phase.

The key is being consistent. These promises go out of the window if you're dabbling with a bit of this, a bit of that and a few glasses of wine here and there. Make up your mind to succeed: decide to start once and just not stop, and to achieve long-lasting results for good.

RESULTS THAT LAST A LIFETIME

For the radical results of my Method to last a lifetime, you need to protect and improve your metabolism and make sure that you change your habits for good.

Motivation is what makes you embark on the programme, but no matter what your personality, that will only last so long. It's the habits that keep you going. As we go through the plan, your focus must be 'I'm changing my habits for good' and not 'I'm on a diet'. This is one of the most important points of my approach, so please don't gloss over it – it'll make the difference between a permanent life change and a terrific but temporary transformation. I want more than a transformation for you – I want it to last forever.

Following a lifestyle that drops body fat, preserves precious muscle mass and drives further toning means that you protect and boost your metabolic rate. Your metabolism is solely driven by how much muscle mass you have in your body (which is why men's calorific needs are greater than women's), and so the more strength you protect and build, the better your metabolism.

In 20 years I've never met a client with a 'bad metabolism' – just bodies that are under-exercised or stripped of muscle through constant dieting. You build this up again by following my protein-rich diet and workout regime. With the right approach, every body can recover and transform. Keep focused on the precision of my Method and on envisioning your 'fat-burning tap' drip-drip-dripping as you protect your metabolism like gold dust.

Even if you have a history of fad dieting and a preconception that results must equal pain, suffering and discomfort, what you are about to experience is anything but – and you'll soon see for yourself that consistency, not severity, will deliver the most astounding results; and that the change itself is as aspirational as the end result you achieve.

Aim high; don't settle for a result that is a compromise, because with my Method you don't need to compromise. You only live once, so you might as well do it in the best body and health you can.

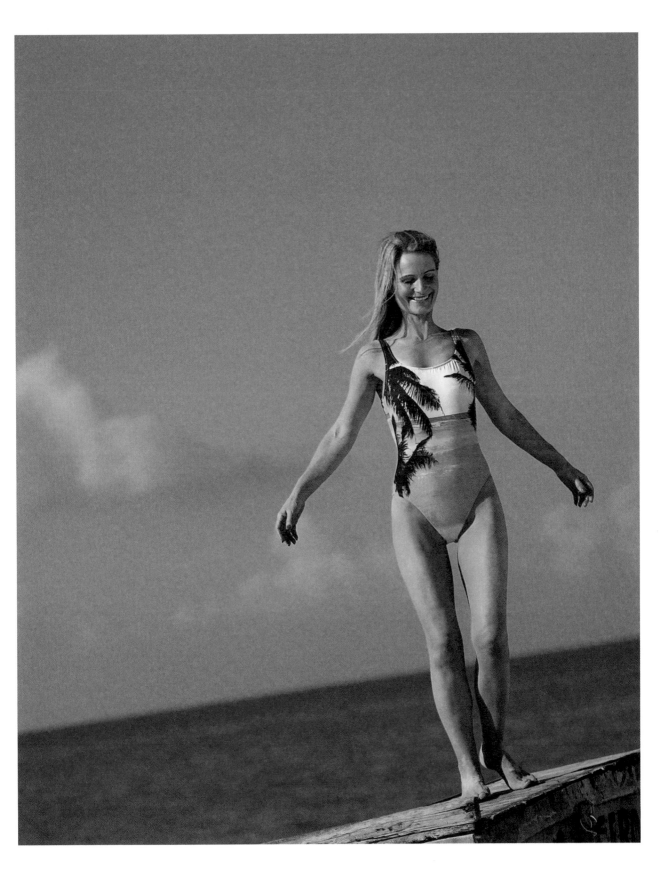

THE VICIOUS CIRCLE OF FAD 'DIETING'

Remember: it is habits that keep you going and enable you to maintain your results. We're going to create new positive habits and let go of the negative ones. Top of the list is to get out of the mad, crazy, soul-destroying cycle of pointless 'fad diets'. Set yourself free – it was the best thing I ever did for myself.

Any 'diet' that is extreme, or deficient in protein or calories, will steal precious muscle and will dehydrate you – showing an impressive 'weight loss' that fools you into thinking it's been a success.

There are two questions to ask yourself before you start any programme:

★ Can I see myself doing 80 per cent of it in five years' time?

★ Would I want my teenage daughter to follow it?

If, deep down, you realize that the answer to either is 'no', don't even go there.

A YEAR OF WEIGHT LOSS

You'll soon see at first hand that a 'weight loss' of 10lb with my Method (which is 10lb of pure fat) has a radically more impressive result than a 'weight loss' of the same amount on a fad diet (where perhaps only one-third is actually fat). Here's a story that might sound familiar.

Let's say it's January, you weigh 150lb, you're fed up that you're one dress size up on last year and so you attempt a two-week juice fast. It's hellish, but you're thrilled to lose 10lb. You now weigh 140lb, but don't fit into your smaller clothes, even though you were 140lb when you wore them last summer. Sadly, your tumble dryer is not to blame – but the juice fast is. The majority of the 'weight loss' was water and muscle: let's say you've lost 3lb of fat, 3lb of muscle and 4lb of water.

So you've lost a little bit of fat, but mainly body tone – leaving your metabolism lower and you unable to fit into your smaller clothes. Because the fast comes to a grinding halt, you're left without a plan and feeling ravenous. Your instinct is to overeat and replenish the food you've been deprived of for two weeks. It's likely that you go for calorie-rich foods – not because you are weak, but because it's human nature and part of your survival instinct. To blame yourself and feel remorseful is like blaming a starving child for stealing food. You eat bigger portions and buy a chocolate bar on the way home, without fail.

For the rest of January and February you overeat and put on 7lb of fat, vowing to start a strict detox in March. You now weigh 147lb, so you think you've progressed since January, but are cross with so little progress. You're actually much worse off than you were in January, with 4lb more of fat and 3lb less muscle and a lower metabolism. You're also feeling disappointed that, once more, you've failed to drop a dress size.

In March you start a strict detox. You cut out wheat, meat, dairy, caffeine and a list of other ingredients that a friend at work tells you make you fat. You've a blinding headache for the first week as your body goes into caffeine withdrawal, but this makes you feel virtuous and you confuse it with 'toxins' leaving your body. The plan is restrictive and impossible to do alongside a 'normal' life, and so you give in to a latte and croissant in week three and pack in the whole thing. You've lost 7lb, which you're pleased with as you think you've lost all the weight you put on after the juice fast. You're back to 140lb.

Sadly, because the plan was deficient in protein and you didn't have an ounce of energy with which to exercise, you've lost 3lb of muscle mass again, 3lb of fat and 1lb of water weight. So since January the net result is that you've gained 1lb of fat and lost a staggering 6lb of muscle, despite all the effort of two arduous 'diets' and declined party invitations.

For the rest of March and April you try to eat sensibly, eating clean foods during the week and letting yourself have a couple of meals out and glasses of wine at the weekend. You start training again. You maintain your weight and recover 1lb of the muscle you lost earlier in the year, which is a good thing for your metabolism. But in May you feel that you've been making a decent effort with no results and you hear of a plan on which you can eat whatever you like, as long as you starve yourself twice a week. 'I can do that,' you think, and you're encouraged that it's worked for Mandy in Accounts, who apparently lost 50lb and said it was soooo easy.

You follow this plan for a month and stop, because you gain 2lb. It's 2lb of fat. You know it's because you are eating way too much on the five 'free days', but you're so hungry you can't help yourself. You give it another go until August, committing for another two months. The starvation days are horrible and, because you can't concentrate at work, you have to do them at the weekend and you get fed up of boring your friends with your 'next big diet'. Come Monday, you're ravenous and start to eat 30 per cent more than you did every day when you weren't really trying in April. The excess of calories is just about balanced by the starvation days, and so you lose no weight at all.

You take August off and drink too much rosé at BBQs, envying the girls who are not hiding in cardigans, and vowing that next year you will be thin.

In September you decide to do something 'sensible' this time and join a slimming group and vow to go every week until Christmas. If so many people do it, it must be credible; and a hall full of people exactly like you encourages you. You start off well, counting every cherry tomato and avoiding all 'sins', and lose 4lb in the first month. It's 3lb of fat and 1lb of muscle.

In October you go on holiday and so you have to cut back on food to make up for the 'sin points' of cocktails with Jane, who won't take no for an answer. You spend the days feeling hungry and annoyed that you can't just have a club sandwich by the pool like everyone else. Club sandwiches are your very favourite thing, and deprivation hangs over you like a cloud of self-pity. On the plane home you give in to a Toblerone that was intended for your dad, because your breakfast cereal meant for 'slimmers' has stimulated your appetite with hidden sugar and absolutely no protein yet is well within your points. You eat six pieces of Toblerone and then write off the whole week ahead, because you think you've ruined the entire thing by eating the chocolate.

You vow to go back to your slimming club the following week, but work gets busy and you decide you can do it on your own and save yourself the fee. You gain the 4lb you lost in September and 3lb more, all of which is fat. You're back up to 145lb, have gained 7lb of fat since January and lost 6lb of muscle.

Your metabolism is sluggish because you've lost more than 15 per cent of your total muscle mass, pushing your metabolism down 15 per cent.

You never get round to 'the diet', and you panic a week before Christmas that the dress you bought last December won't do up unless you lie down. You need something quick this time, and so you do a week of high-fat, high-protein food. The weight loss is satisfying, but you can't bear the sight of another egg and fantasize about eating an orange. You lose 4lb that week, half of which is water, half of which is fat.

Christmas arrives and you indulge in everything but are riddled with guilt and don't enjoy your meals. The Christmas roast tastes good, but less wonderful because you've spoilt your appetite eating a chocolate orange, which you didn't even properly enjoy. Your clothes feel tight and you vow that this coming year you are going to really lose weight this time. You're going to become one of those girls on Instagram who post pictures of coconut porridge and goji berries. You gain 3lb of fat over Christmas.

Between Christmas and New Year you trial lots of super-healthy, organic, nourishing recipes with ingredients that your local supermarket doesn't stock, and it feels good to have bee pollen and cocoa nibs in your pantry. You eat coconut porridge for breakfast drenched in the most expensive honey, and yummy brown rice with tofu for lunch in a bento box that you proudly take in to work. In the evening you prepare a huge quinoa salad with two ripe avocados, lots of olive oil and a mass of seeds. You snack on homemade granola bars made with agave nectar, raisins and coconut oil, and it feels so virtuous that you've joined the 'healthy halo' movement.

You weigh yourself on New Year's Eve and are livid that you've gained 2lb, both of which are fat. Whilst the foods you've been eating are nutritious, the diet is dense in calories and suitable for girls who teach four yoga classes a day. Your suppressed metabolism can't take it and you feel baffled as to why it seems to work for everyone but you.

So in a year of dieting and deprivation, you've done a juice fast, a detox, tried intermittent fasting, joined a slimming club, done a week of protein-only and tried hard to be super-organically healthy. You weigh 146lb, which is 4lb less than last January, but you've gained 9lb of fat and lost a staggering 6lb of muscle and 15 per cent of your metabolism.

If this story sounds familiar, then it's time to stop dieting – and start the Louise Parker Method.

IT'S NOT YOU – IT'S THE DIET

In deciding to succeed with my Method, you need to let go of what you perceive as your previous failures with dieting in general. Many diets work for the short period you are doing them, if the sole measure is 'weight loss'. But if the measure is actual fat loss and the longevity of results, then it's a completely different story.

By telling yourself that you always fail, you've tried everything and absolutely nothing works for you, you perpetuate failure. I think it is easier to talk more compassionately to yourself if you genuinely take on board that *you* have not been the failure – it's the diets themselves that have failed you.

I hate crash diets, although I understand that people want results as fast as is humanly possible. But it is possible to achieve this without crash dieting or jumping on the bandwagon of every new diet craze. I don't hide the fact that I loathe juice fasts, which strip away muscle at the most alarming rate and rob you of your metabolism.

Many slimming clubs pay little attention to adequate protein and the balancing of macronutrients (nutritional compounds that are required by the body in large amounts), which is an essential prerequisite for maintaining metabolism and managing appetite. Without this, the dieter fails – and it isn't their fault. The food plans they are congratulated on following literally stimulate their appetite by loading them with low-fat, high-sugar foods. They rely on sheer willpower alone, whilst appetites rage; and it's no surprise to me that their long-term failure rate is 80 per cent.

I think physiological 'detoxing' is all a bit dubious unless you're coming off heroin, and I've never really understood what 'toxins' people are detoxing from. If you fundamentally change your diet long-term, your body will come into excellent health and you won't need to cleanse it. Just start to eat beautifully and your body will take care of itself.

I've made all these mistakes myself and I truly understand how it feels to be desperate, but I also know that there is a simpler, more intelligent, scientific and a far kinder way – with results that absolutely wipe the floor of any crash diet.

LEARN LEAN

I'm going to get you a body that is defined and glowing – you at your very, very best. You'll be healthy, fit and lean. It's all too easy to confuse these three things, and it matters because each one is so very different.

Barely a day goes by without a new scientific study exclaiming the benefits of drinking a glass of red wine or eating dark chocolate every day. It might be good for your health, and your blood pressure might thank you, but your behind won't shrink.

And whilst coconut and cocoa nibs are full of 'goodness', don't be fooled: they're often so calorific that they're working against you, if you're trying to look good on the beach. So 'good' are the calories in the raw-food trend that we've seen a massive increase in clients who are following these diets and are now 'organically overweight'.

With the exercise you'll be doing every day you'll get fitter, and so you can forget talk of 'fit, not skinny'. You're going to be 'fit *and* lean'.

So the confusion stops here, and I promise I will show you not just the healthy way, but the lean way and – most importantly – the sustainable way.

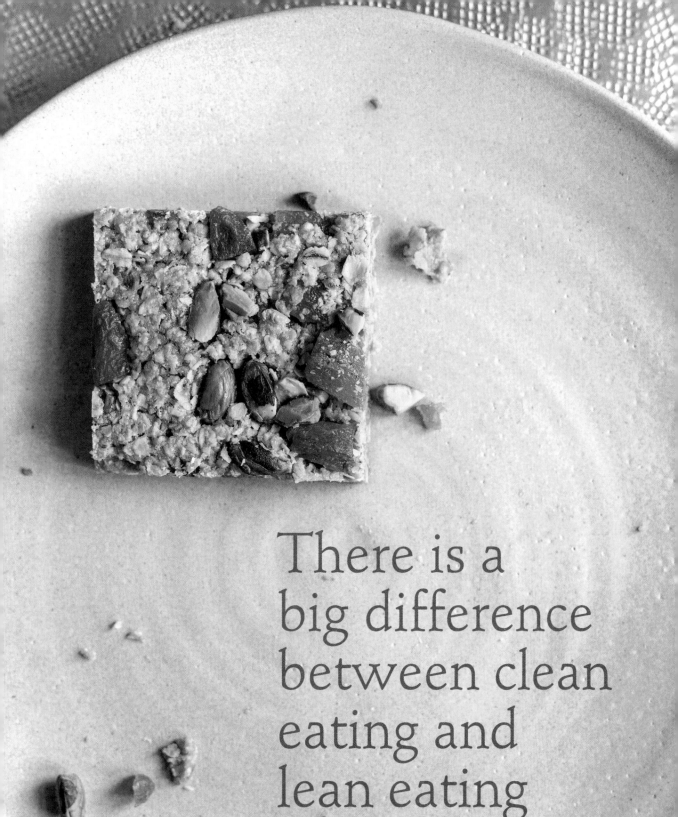

There is a
big difference
between clean
eating and
lean eating

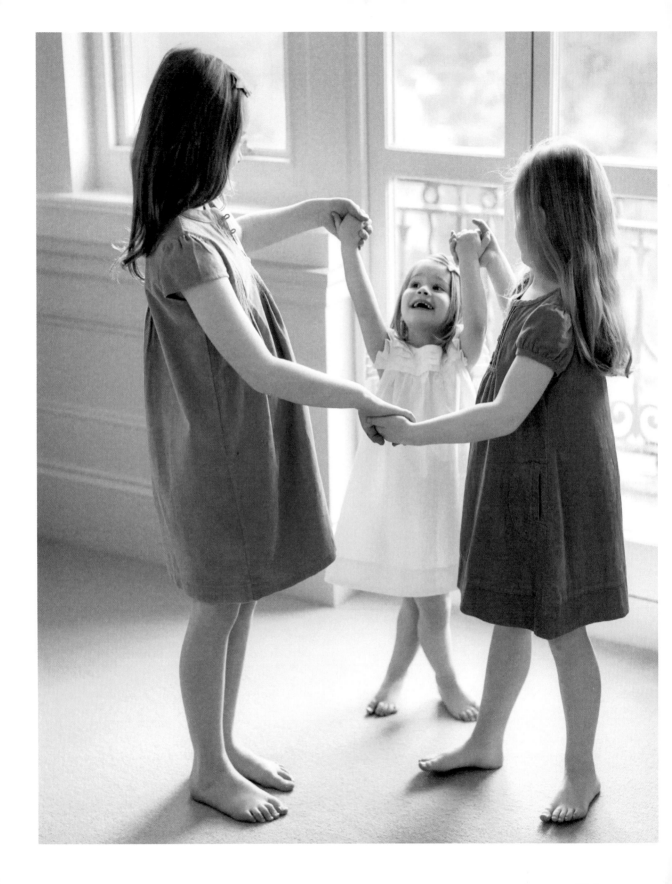

THE DANCE

Think of my Method as a sort of dance that, when you learn the steps and practise, will become part of who you are, and not something you are 'doing'. When you arrive at your goal, you're going to be in the habit of eating beautifully most of the time, but will also celebrate in perfect balance, without a hint of guilt and always so that your dress size no longer fluctuates.

Imagine an inner circle (which represents the core of the Method that you aim to follow 100 per cent of the time in the Transform Phase), surrounded by an outer circle. Before you start the programme I will help you to define what being in this inner circle means, breaking down your goal into bite-sized pieces.

Throughout your programme you'll stay bang in the middle of the inner circle until you reach your goal. As your transformation progresses there will be times when it feels so easy to stay in this inner circle; but you'll also probably have moments that test you. When this happens, visualize the inner circle and stay focused that your one job is to remain inside it. Try not to step outside it, and don't let anyone push you out. Be stubborn, be determined, be proud and really focus on staying inside the circle.

If you do pop out of the inner circle (a glass of wine, a biscuit or two, a day or two of missed exercise), do not panic. Falling out of the circle is not the end of the world. Simply jump straight back into the inner circle, as your aim is to spend as much time as possible here.

You're ending 'stinking thinking' (see page 31) and the habits that sabotage results, so I don't want you to think that the biscuit has ruined the whole thing – I want you always to come home again to the inner circle. Think of it as getting a cab home after a couple of drinks, rather than catching a flight to Vegas for a three-day party.

The more time you spend in the inner circle and the less time in the outer circle, the sooner you will 'get the habit' and reach your goal. Remember: the easiest route is the direct route.

You'll stay in this inner circle every day until you reach your goal. Armed with your fabulous results, you can now start to dance in the outer circle (a Sunday roast, half a bottle of wine with friends), but you always pop back into the inner circle, where you'll spend about 80 per cent of your time. I cringe when I hear anyone say that they 'cheated'; drinking a glass of wine isn't cheating – it's just a step in the dance.

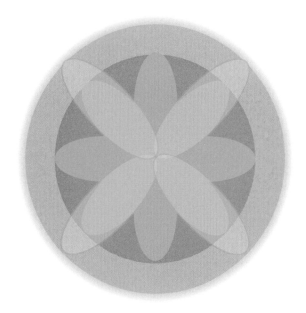

Depending on how active you are, you'll probably spend about 20 per cent of your time in the outer circle. But you step out, step back, step out, step home – you don't spend four days at home and three days out. That's not balance: that's 'on' and 'off' behaviour – and there's a big difference.

Of course there will be times of the year when it makes sense for you to step outside both circles, and it would be weird and too restrictive not to. At Christmas, New Year, your birthday weekend in Paris, where all your meals are a celebration and your exercise routine gets put to one side. It'll happen occasionally, and most likely it will be 'worth it'. Enjoy it – just don't do it too often.

I go without nothing that I really crave or desire on holiday, or in life in general. If I want it, I have it – and dance straight back into the inner circle. It's become such a habit that I don't even have to think about it. I love the true freedom of the dance. But like all new dance moves, you need to learn the steps until they become your natural rhythm.

1

★ Adopt a positive mindset and assume success
★ Make time for simple pleasures every single day
★ Deal with and dissolve all your worries
★ Keep positive, inspiring company

THIINK SUCCESSFULLY

The mindset part of my Method is the first and probably the most important of the four pillars. You're going to cultivate a winning mindset and repeat it until it becomes a habit. The brain is the most important muscle in your transformation, and you are going to train it consistently, as you would your body.

For my own personal development, and in committing myself to ensuring that each Louise Parker client reaches their full potential, I have somewhat obsessively tried to understand the mindset of winners. Talent, strategy and preparation clearly pave the way, but it's when these things collide with an absolute expectation of success that brilliance is born. Whether you're a premiership footballer, the CEO of a FTSE 100 company or are simply trying to lose weight – you need the same ingredients to win. Apply the execution that a premiership footballer would to making the England squad, or a businesswoman to becoming CEO, to the pursuit of permanent weight loss – and you will succeed. Think of it as a business plan for your body: you have a clear vision, a strategy to execute the plan, inputs and outputs,

company values and a culture of thinking, and the result is a successful business. Your body is no different.

My clients have usually realized infinite achievements, with their body being the missing link – and my role is to coach them in the habits of permanent health. Part of my job is directing the same principles of success that they apply to other areas of their lives to the four pillars of my Method, and then it all falls beautifully into place.

What I want is for you to adopt the habit of a positive mindset that strives for excellence. This isn't to be confused with perfection, which does not exist; but simply that you strive for the best version of yourself that you can – in mind and body.

We want to create the habit of thinking positively. Every time your mind veers towards 'stinking thinking' (see page 31), you are going to pull it back and replace it with a positive outlook. At first it will feel peculiar, as it would driving on the wrong side of the road. But the more you do it – day in, day out – and keep turning your thoughts around, the more it will become your New Normal.

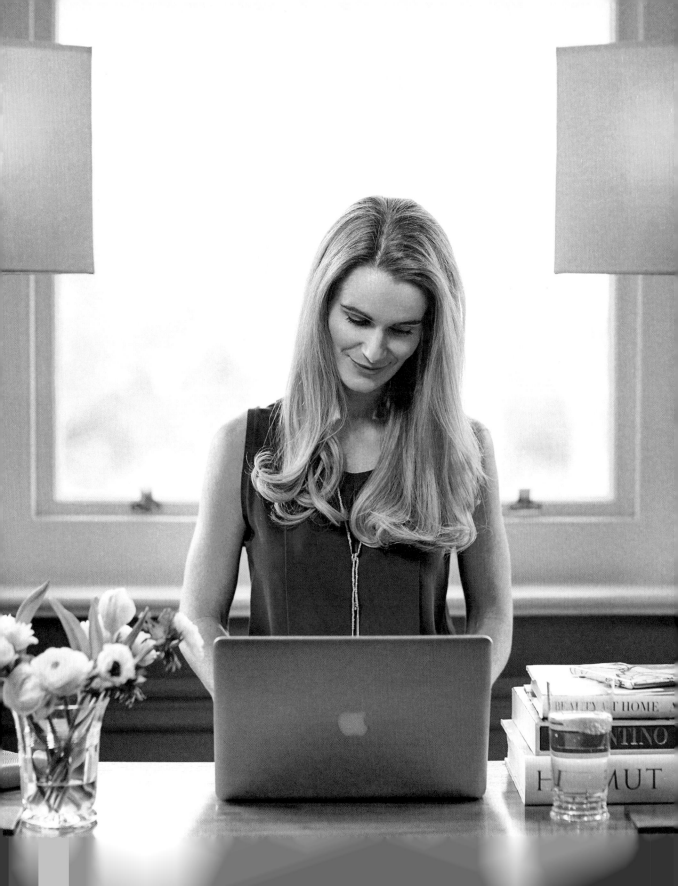

Don't Do It – Become It

When you get the habit of excellence, it will become part of who you are. As long as the lifestyle you're trying to attain is separate from you – like juices being delivered to your door for seven days, a slimming-club programme you say you are doing 'until I lose 20 pounds' or a detox that you go on for three days – it will not last. It will always remain separate from you and will never become part of who you are. Think of my Method as an anti-diet: you're learning how to get forever habits in the real world.

The Louise Parker Method goes beyond something that you are 'doing at the moment' – it is 'just what you do' and, when this happens, it becomes lasting change. As you start, it will of course feel like something new and possibly challenging, as you readjust your habits of eating, sleeping, training and thinking. Approach these changes as steps in a new dance, and not with a 'diet' mentality, which will always come to a grinding halt. Remember: you are achieving permanent change and ending trend dieting for good.

Why do millions achieve radical and life-changing weight loss and then put it all back on again? Isn't it galling that the business models of the world's most popular slimming clubs are based on failure, and that the vast majority of customers return time and again when they put the weight back on? It's my belief that as long as the person 'doing it' feels they are separate from it – white-knuckling it, ignoring the necessity to make the plan a lifestyle – they will always stop. Because everything that remains something that you 'do', with a start date and an end date, and that is separate from you, you will eventually 'stop'. Even more so when the conditions are unsustainable, as they usually are. Think beyond the end date of Transform. The six-week programme will deliver you fabulous results, but it is intended to recalibrate your habits so that the last day in fact becomes the first day of your New Normal. Day 42 is not the end of a programme, but the start of a new way of living.

Ensuring the Perfect Fit for You

For the Louise Parker Method to become a part of you, it needs to fit you beautifully. Whilst the Method is precise, there is choice, and you'll need to 'find your perfect fit' to truly suit you. If it feels like a pair of Spanx, loosen it a little until it's comfortable. It's about finding a comfort level that is sustainable for you.

If you like to train at nine at night, do that. The best time to train every day is the time that it will actually happen every day. If you don't like something, don't eat it – it will never become a habit. Explore your favourite food options; put effort into finding habits that will continually punctuate your day with an 'Aaaaah'. You'll need a repertoire of meals that suit you and your family and that suit your lifestyle.

We're aiming for you to eat to this style 80 per cent of the time for ever – and for ever is a really long time. If you're serious about permanent habit change, then you really need to think about this point and find what fits you so beautifully that you'll want to always wear it.

For my Method to become part of you, it needs to fit beautifully. It's about a comfort level that's sustainable

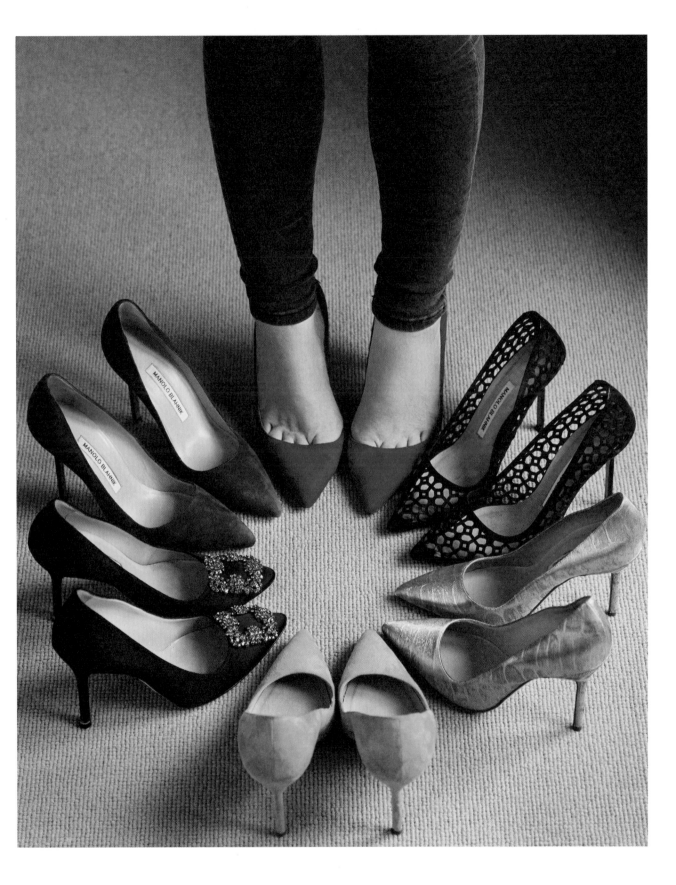

Be Bold

The Method is about aiming high and reaching your absolute potential, and this requires being bold. You'll need to be bold in attitude, actions and aspiration as you kick off your programme. As impressive results come your way, which they will, you'll want to continue with gusto. It starts with a bit of hope, a leap of faith, which I'm going to help you cultivate into a winning mindset. You have to sprout that first blossom of bold determination and I'll help you to nurture it, but you will have to tend it every day for it to grow.

If you start half-heartedly, neglect the preparation or set a goal that just doesn't excite you, you'll risk mediocrity, and my Method is not about mediocrity – it's about pulling something really special out of the bag.

Don't leave any of it to luck, or expect something extraordinary from putting in something ordinary. No one has a great body due to luck. I agree that there are some bodies that are created to model and be swooned over – many of which I have worked with. What I do know is that modelling has become more about looking healthy, fit and glowing and less about scrawny 'heroin chic'. Most of the highly successful models train and eat like athletes. They'd look pretty good if they did nothing, but not good enough to model, and I promise that if they sat about eating badly, they'd gain weight.

They may gain weight slower than you and I, but an unhealthy lifestyle always, always catches up with you.

I don't believe in luck – which I suppose is strange, for a girl who met her husband at baggage reclaim. Paul was never meant to be on my flight from Hong Kong to London, but having missed his flight from Shanghai had to take an unexpected detour. We'd stood 10ft apart for no more than ten minutes, waiting for our luggage, when his bags arrived and he walked away. Something inside me stirred – a boldness I've never felt before – and I swiftly followed him and tapped him on the shoulder. I've never done that before or since, I might add. I often think about how that rare moment of boldness changed the course of my life, and how my split-second decision created this remarkable life and family that we share. I still don't think it was luck – just a bold decision that happened to go my way. Fortune does indeed favour the brave.

I'd like you to be bold in your decision to take on each and every pillar of my Method and to expect nothing but success. Remember that you are aiming to achieve something you've never done before, and so you need to be bolder than you've ever been before. Be bold in all of it – your decision to start, your positivity, your workouts, your meals, your enthusiasm, your expectation.

Know Your Strategy & Don't Pick-and-Mix

My Method is the optimum strategy for succeeding at permanent weight loss and health. Everything I give you in each of the four pillars comes together in one strategy that cannot fail, if you work at it. Make sure you understand the whys and whens – you'll apply yourself more fully when you truly understand them. Don't pick-and-mix a bit of my Method with a bit of another – the strategy is carefully calibrated to make the journey as easy and effective as possible. It's a judicious balance, which can be tipped by introducing another system. If there was anything else that I could add to make it more effective, I would have done so. It's all here, so don't change a recipe that's tried and tested – and that really works.

Define your goals, bin them and think again, this time 30 per cent bolder

Dream a Bigger Dream

To succeed in anything you need to have clear objectives and a clear strategy. The same goes for my Method. You need to define what your objectives are, to power the strategy that the Louise Parker Method provides.

You need to define success – what does it mean to you? All I ask is that you define it, bin it and think again, this time 30 per cent bolder. No one in their right mind is going to make a daily commitment to mediocrity, so dream a bigger dream. Your goals need to excite you and boldly propel you into the programme, until the habits fall into place.

Given that we've got a strategy that works beautifully, why not make your goals greater than you've ever aimed for previously? There is not a single body that cannot morph into something beautifully strong, lean, slender, elegant and ridiculously healthy. It would defy science to follow my Method and not achieve a thrilling result. If you've got a longer journey, it will simply take a little longer, but the time will pass anyway.

You become what you think about, so carefully choose your thoughts, which become what you say. Your words become your actions and habits, which create the body and the life you aim for. Don't sell yourself short. And don't play lip service to your dream, because your heart must believe it. We call it 'placing your order'. Dig deep and dig in, because you deserve an abundant life, in the healthiest, happiest and most beautiful body.

Visualize Victory in the Movies of Your Mind

Visualizing your goal is paramount to success and I love the saying 'going to the movies of your mind'. Your victory needs to be defined, precise and tangible, so that you can feel it when you close your eyes. You should literally feel a warmth, a tingle down your spine. Don't even think about not succeeding.

Take one teeny hour to create *your* vision in the 'movies of your mind', and go beyond the aesthetic – it'll mean the difference between smashing your goals and mediocrity. Think about how you will *feel* in your body, rather than what you *look like* in your body. You have to feel it, not just see it. When you feel powerful, lean, strong and self-assured, I can assure you that you are going to look hot in your body.

I can still feel the vision I created for myself when I was about to begin my second post-natal transformation, when Milly was a few months old. I'd decided to regain my body in time for a holiday to Thailand, 12 weeks away. I didn't even for a minute think that I would *not* achieve it. I placed my order, visualized it and assumed it would happen.

I had 14kg (30lb) to drop, a body to tone back to strength, and two children who didn't sleep. I would not, however, be deterred. I remember placing my order on a bracing walk on Wimbledon Common. I could feel myself standing on the first step of an infinity pool, with Sophie playing contentedly in the water beside me and Milly upon my hip, her little chubby legs hanging between the strings of my white bikini. My body is warm, my skin tingling from the sunshine and the water is cool beneath me. There's the smell of hot ground that rises after a monsoon rainfall. I feel content, poised and powerful in my body.

I kept taking my mind back to this single moment, time and again, until three months later I actually stood there. I had the most powerful sense of déjà vu – which shouldn't have been surprising, as I'd mentally experienced this moment a hundred times already. Visualization is so very powerful that the brain can't really distinguish between the imagined and reality. Your brain literally builds the pathways that it will recall as a route to make your visualization a reality.

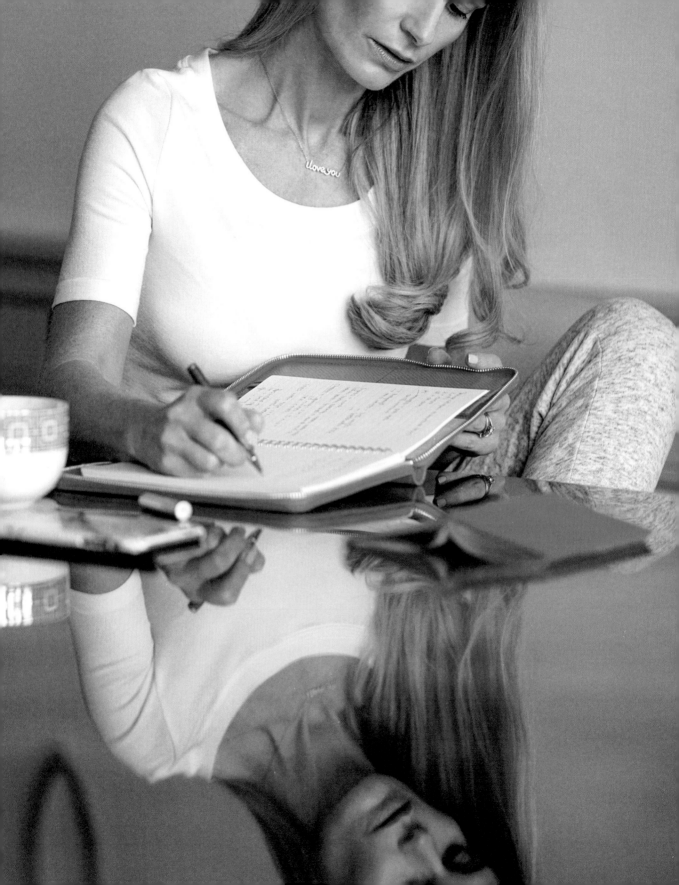

Ink It – Don't Think It

It's not a clear goal until it is written down. I love the maxim 'Think in Ink' and am forever writing down my goals. For your visualization to become reality, take the time to commit it to paper. You'll improve your results by defining your visualized goals in ink, allowing them to connect with the rest of the programme. Remember to define what success means to you – far beyond 'I want to lose weight'. Write down the visualization that you're going to take your mind to, over the coming weeks. Make a list of five other goals, which will get your pulse racing and motivate you through any challenging moments.

Start Once & Just Don't Stop

Now is always a good time to start. There will never be a six-week period in your life free of travel, weddings, events and projects.

Throughout the Transform Phase you're going to follow every single strategy, to the very best you can, every single day. I am 100 per cent convinced that the direct route is by far the easiest route. For a decade we've run programmes at my company that take our clients directly to their goal – no faffing about. It's consistency that forms the habit. And habit that wins the race. You need to make a decision to start once and just not stop, no matter what – until you reach your goal. Nothing can steer you off-course from your goals unless you allow it to.

Anticipate each hurdle, vocalize it with your friends, decide how you will leap over it and report back. Being accountable is one of the greatest powers behind 'Starting Once'. Having done the programme at full throttle three times, after the birth of all my daughters, I know how powerful this is; I reported in weekly to a member of my team, knowing that doing so would increase my results significantly and make the journey easier.

When the going gets tough, read your goals, phone a friend or, best of all, get outside and walk – and go to the 'movies of your mind'. If you fall down, learn how to get straight back up again, rather than reverting to 'stinking thinking' and writing a whole week off. Don't allow a packet of Maltesers to turn into a week of overeating, when you can start again at the very next meal. The difference between getting this habit and *not* getting this habit is fundamental to change.

Don't confuse 'treating myself with a day off' with a treat. What you're doing instead is unravelling four days' work and going in the opposite direction from your goals. It's a bit like doing a four-day spring-clean and then letting teenagers throw a house party – absolutely pointless, and you've now got to spend another four days tidying up.

Reward yourself with things that make you feel fabulous and have absolutely nothing to do with food: clear out your wardrobe, redesign your living room, deal with an issue that is eating away at you – anything that will make you feel better. This does of course take concentration, and perhaps even a level of healthy obsession.

Healthy Obsession

The word 'obsession' is tricky. You're aiming to find another way of living and get off the roller coaster of trend dieting, and you also want fabulous results. So I'm going to rid you of the obsession of 'dieting' and 'not dieting', and all the baggage it brings with it – both physical and emotional.

The rewards for consistency during Transform are the results you'll achieve and the habits you'll form – both of which will free you from the obsession of dieting. To gain freedom from this obsession, a level of healthy obsession in staying the course is required, to enable the consistency to do its magic. When you are consistent, habits are created.

So a degree of healthy obsession is no bad thing; it will get you to your goal and glue the habits in place. Whether it's healthy obsession or total dedication, it is what sets you apart from those who may never cross the finish line.

Every 'winner' that I've met to date has had a level of obsession that they have cultivated in a positive way to achieve a desired outcome. Don't spend your Sunday afternoons preparing a week's worth of Tupperware meals; that's just depressing and won't last. But do think ahead and plan – just make it sensible, sustainable and keep in mind that we're building habits that must last the five-year test.

See the Obstacle & Leap Over It

Once you've turned on the switch in your mind, no obstacle is insurmountable and you'll get into the habit of steering around problems, each swerve boosting your motivation.

When you see challenges as exciting and a positive exercise in accountability, it positively changes your focus and results. Know that there will be parties, and moments when you will doubt your determination. Decide that in these moments you will 'stay in the circle' anyway. When you keep thinking of stepping outside the circle, pull your mind back and don't allow it to go there. Don't let your mind feed the doubtful or negative thoughts.

See the mental challenge as exciting, and prove to yourself how strong your mind is. You have no idea how mentally strong you can be until you ask it of yourself.

On the eve of starting my final post-natal transformation, I went for a hike on the Sussex Downs and made the decision to start once and just not stop, until I reached my goal. I knew it was a really challenging time to start but that timing is never perfect. I was bleeding from the eyeballs with tiredness, juggling work and a newborn, and had a stream of weekend guests to stay, to ogle over my delicious new baby. They were tough times, but good times. The toughest was going to be the annual fortnight when my two brothers and I join families at our house in Sussex for a string of summer days spent idling away in conversation on the lawn and drinking Pimm's – usually a lot of it.

I made my decision to step over it and still enjoy it. I'd train every day before anyone woke up, and simply cooked all the delicious food from my plan for everyone. We feasted on fruit platters and Bircher muesli for breakfast, marinated grilled chicken and divine salads for lunch, and steaks and legs of lamb in the evening, with spring vegetables from the garden. I cooked grilled nectarines and peaches, served with passion fruit Greek yogurt and mint. I made new potato salad and bought fresh brown bread rolls for the table, which I simply skipped; it was no big deal, as I loved the food I was eating. I passed on the wine and Pimm's, which was a challenge for sure. That fortnight I dropped 3kg (6½lb) and had such a magical summer. With hindsight I've never once thought that a few glasses of rosé or a handful of new potatoes would've improved it. I proved to myself that no situation or obstacle is insurmountable. Don't work obstacles up to prevent you from starting – just start.

Consistency, Not Severity

Throughout the Transform Phase you're going to stick consistently to the habits of the Method, every day, performing them over and over again until they stick. By repeating the strategies of success time and again, you'll get your body to achieve marginal gains from all the four pillars, every day – resulting in phenomenal transformation.

We will turn our backs on any form of severity and create a lifestyle that fits so comfortably that you can wear it well, most of the time, for ever.

During the Lifestyle Plan, consistency relaxes into an approach whereby you continue to live with beautiful habits for the most part, but you can afford to eat with celebration when it's 'worth it' to you, without compromising your amazing new body. You can have it all.

By practising consistency in all of the pillars, you build habits that last a lifetime and work towards your goal, inch by inch. Results will come fabulously fast when you find a pace that you can stick at – where the 'fat-burning tap' just keeps drip-drip-dripping.

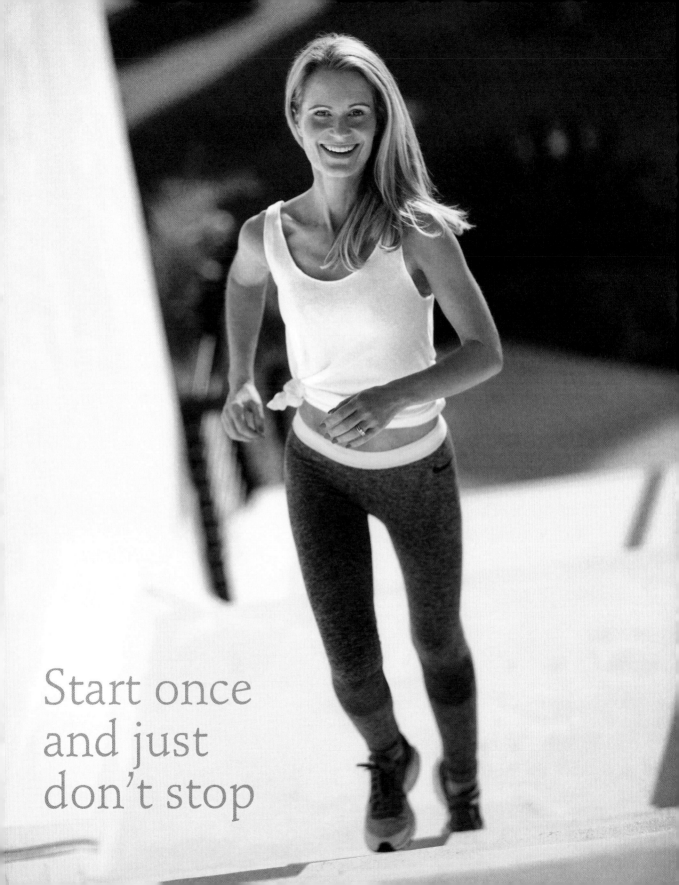

Start once
and just
don't stop

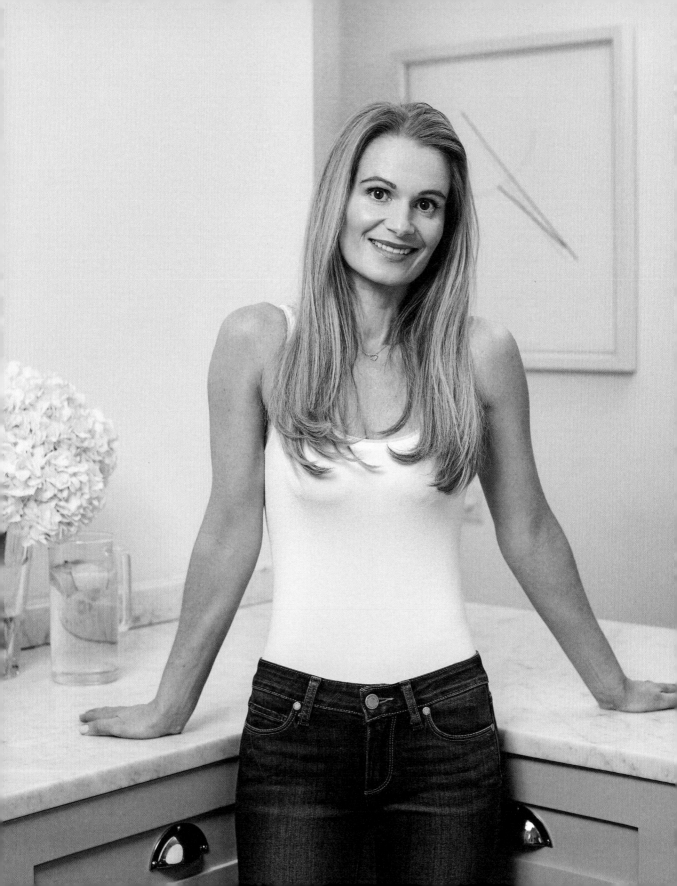

Perfection Does Not Exist

I know how crippling it can be to be a perfectionist and I'm not suggesting that, alongside your determination, you apply the pressure of perfectionism. Perfection does not exist. Everyone will have a blip – maybe even a handful of them. Just get straight back up again at the very next meal. See a hiccup as an opportunity to revisit your targets and come back stronger; and always remember that you can start your day again at any point. Turn it around the very next minute, put it behind you and crack on.

Imperfection is not failure – it is just a reality of the ebb and flow of life. So whilst you focus on being determined, don't see a blip or indiscretion as the end of the world. It does not mean that you won't achieve incredible results. It's about recognizing that consistency is an integral part of the strategy, so you don't have to be severe – it won't collapse if you are not perfect. But do be as consistent as you can.

Don't sabotage progress by thinking that if you've not nailed each day with perfection you might as well sod it, write off the next few days and 'start again on Monday'. This is where perfectionism can lead to 'fat thinking'. You wouldn't get sunburned and think: 'Sod it, I'm going to cover myself in baby oil and lie in the midday sun.'

Recognize Stinking Thinking

It's by recognizing and tossing away 'stinking thinking' that the strategy of your lifestyle habits, eating habits and workout habits will come together. First, you need to recognize the thoughts that keep you at arm's length from succeeding in making a true lifestyle change. Let go of past failures and leave them where they are – in the past. Give up the 'on it' and 'off it' diet mentality, and be accountable for the excuses you've been using to avoid success. I've never actually met a client with a 'bad metabolism' – simply lower muscle mass, which can be increased. Make sure that you have not been more scared of succeeding than of losing, because that's a familiar place to sit.

Write down your negative thoughts and decide on the positive swaps that you need to make.

Fake it Till You Make it

You'll have heard this a thousand times, but believe it. Act like the person you want to become. Adopt the habits, walk the walk, think the thoughts and become the better version of yourself. Faking it until you make the habits is sometimes essential to get you going. I'm rarely nervous, with the two exceptions being flying and public speaking, both of which are essential parts of my life. I've tried everything: hypnotism, meditation and even medication.

The only solution that works is faking it. I simply pretend that I love public speaking and that I'm the world's greatest public speaker – and acting like that girl just for a moment kicks me off to get me going. I do the same on a flight – at take-off I pretend that I love the exhilaration of taking off and that the feeling in my stomach is actually the anticipation of adventure. It works every time.

Place your order for results that will truly astound you

We Are Better Together

Undeniably, in teams and with support, we achieve greater things. I've experienced this in so many areas of my life. The success of my company is entirely down to a team effort – everyone making an excellent contribution to the sum of its parts. I believe anything is possible if a team shares the same values and goals. Our signature programmes at Louise Parker rely on all the strategies of the Method, along with constant support, no matter where in the world our clients are.

Sharing, honesty, motivation and being accountable are all essential ingredients for success. So do ask another person, or a gaggle, to join you – if you are together, incredible things will happen. You will do better together, so don't avoid it because it requires a bit more effort. It could make the difference between achieving the body of your dreams and a lifestyle that lasts, and not quite reaching them. Pick up the phone and ask a friend or three to join you.

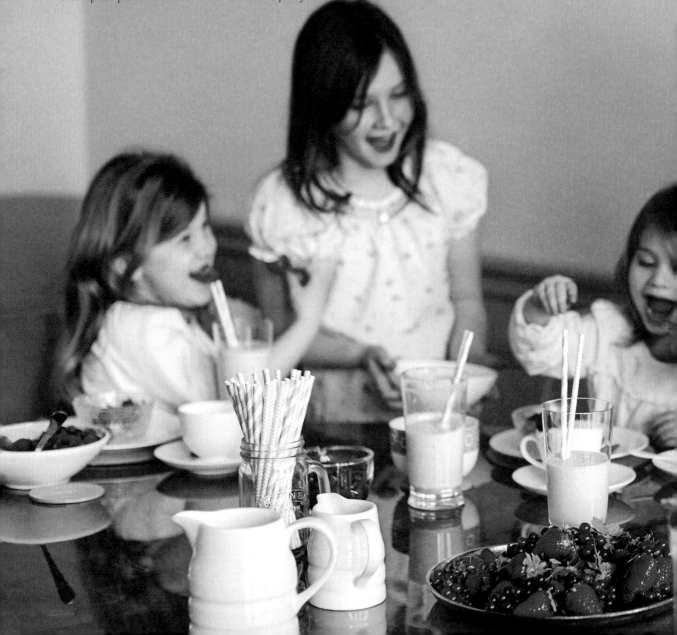

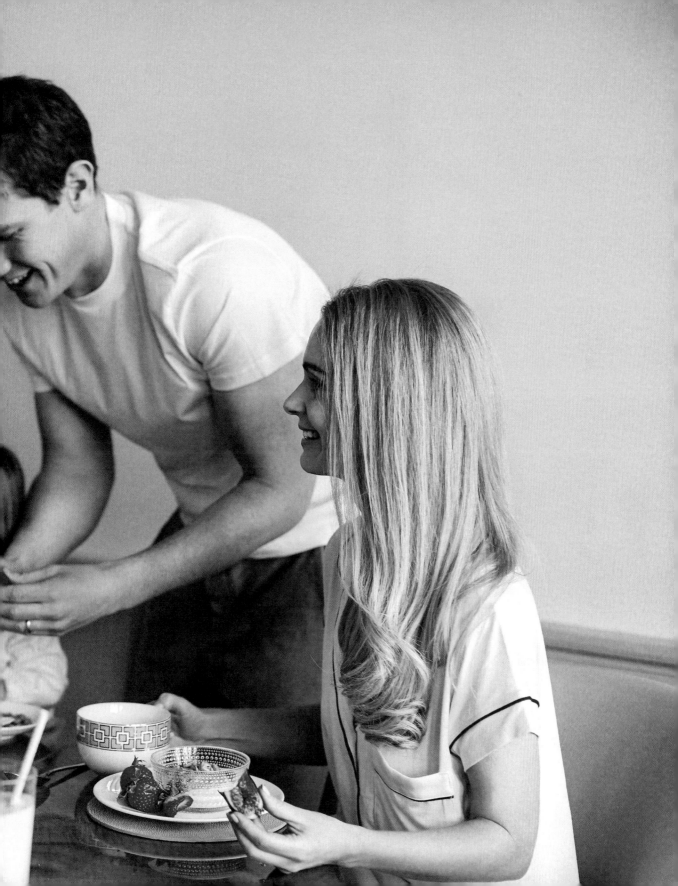

2

★ Declutter your surroundings
★ Digital detox after 9pm every night
★ Sleep 7 hours a night
★ Take a 'brain-nap' for 20 minutes a day

LIVE WELL

In this section you'll create lifestyle habits that really make you feel good. They have both a scientific and a feel-good purpose, and they form the glue that makes the other three pillars stand the test of time. You'll create them during the Transform Phase, but you'll also need to tend to them as you ease into the Lifestyle Plan – nurturing them so that your life and body continually improve.

It's essential that you face into your stress and your sleeping habits, as they impact upon the hormones that support weight loss. You will learn how to replace clutter, chaos, dread and disorganization with a prepared, ordered and serene lifestyle, so that you achieve a life that feels so beautiful, you'll never want to go back to where you were previously.

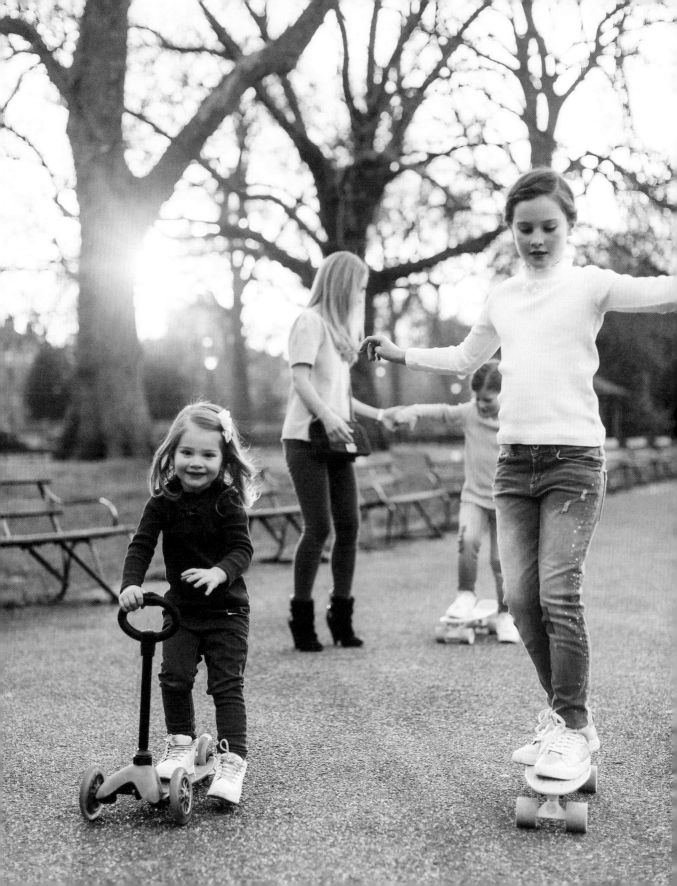

Beautiful Surroundings

You're going to make your surroundings beautiful.

I believe in making everything that surrounds you as beautiful as you can – whether it's your bedside table, your place setting, your workout space or your desk – because it impacts on your mood, motivation and mindset in the most profoundly positive way.

The first step of Transform is to prepare and pave the way for a calm, organized path to success. You'll do this before you start. So there may be a push in the first few days of the programme, but you will need to keep tending to it and pulling out the weeds that threaten your serenity.

If any of these improvements are big tasks, take the time to visualize it, think it, ink it and set aside the time to do it. No lifestyle is going to feel beautiful, relaxed and calm amongst mess and chaos, so don't overlook this, as an exercise in potpourri.

★ Declutter your surroundings and get rid of objects that are neither practical nor beautiful. Your home and work space should reflect the way you feel about yourself.

★ Keep a beautifully stocked and clean fridge, larder, freezer and kitchen, investing in gorgeous storage that makes everything quicker and easier to find and a pleasure to look at.

★ Surround yourself with objects that you love, wherever you spend the most time – photographs that lift your mood, a framed note from a child, a single flower in a glass.

★ Prepare a calm space in your home to work out in, and make sure it's a place that *feels* good: you should be able to transform it into your home gym in two minutes. I train in my sitting room with a few pieces of kit stored in a beautiful box behind the door.

★ Consistently keep track of bills and admin so that you never have to 'spring-clean' and don't get bogged down in stress, but instead adopt a 'Do it Now' attitude. I wish I'd learned this two decades ago.

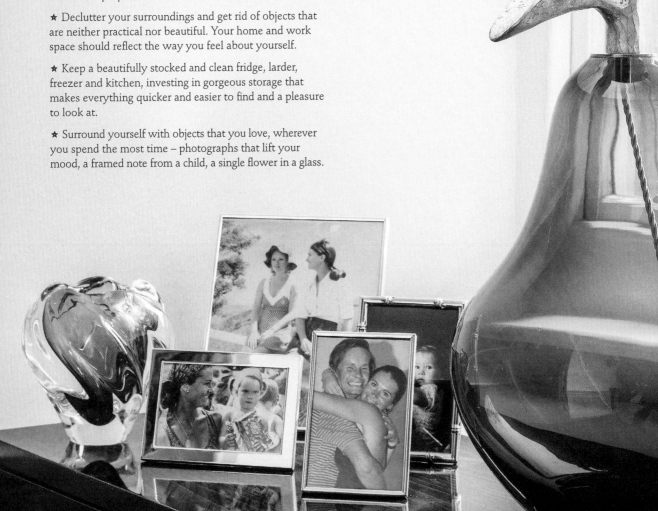

Eating with Style

You're going to eat 'with celebration' and style.

In the Eat Beautifully chapter (see page 50) you'll find
80 recipes that form the basis of my Method. They are
all designed to be inspiring, beautiful and, most of all,
deliciously simple. But how you prepare and eat them is
as important as the ingredients themselves. Take a few
extra minutes to make your meals look as gorgeous as you
can; 'eating with ceremony' – no matter how simple your
snack – is part of eating beautifully. It reminds you that
you are 'worth it'. It will encourage you to fall in love
with your beautiful style of eating, which is a lifestyle
commitment that will last for ever. No more eating at
the fridge. That's not chic.

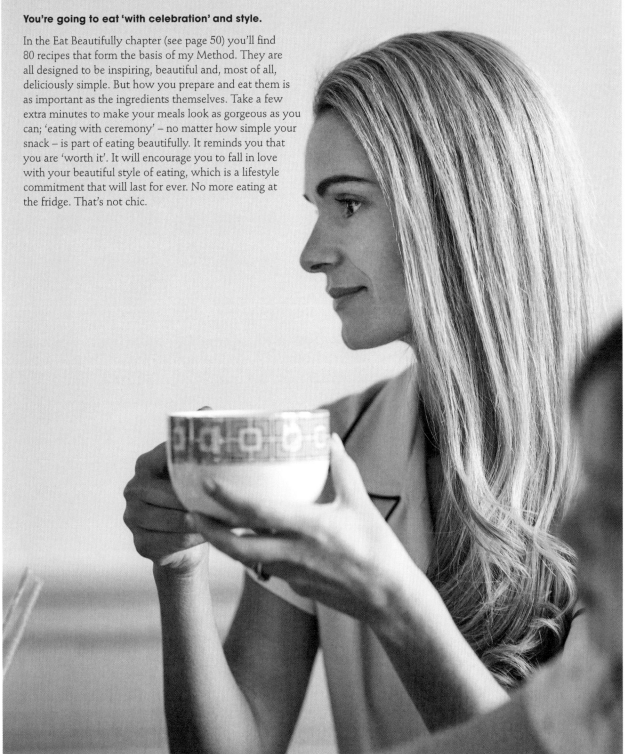

Sleep, Sleep, Sleep

You're going to sleep for seven hours a night, and super-sleep when you can.

Your short-term and long-term results will be staggeringly improved when you adjust your lifestyle to enhance the quality and duration of your sleep. We're going to get your bedtime routine and sleep into a regular pattern and ensure that you get seven hours' sleep every night. On weeks where there are unavoidable obstacles, you'll catch up with a 'super-sleep' over the weekend. It just requires a little shuffling of your routine for the first few weeks until it becomes normal.

I'd say that about half of our clients come to us suffering from some sort of sleep disorder – whether it's constant deprivation, not being able to get to sleep, waking in the night or being woken early by a child. If a client is TATT (tired all the time), we have to fix it fast.

Lack of sleep is a profound contributory factor in fat gain and simply has to be tackled, for longevity of results. If you are sleep-deprived, your fat loss will slow down – and you'll find maintaining your results a battle.

Sleep helps weight loss by regulating the function of hormones that directly correlate to appetite and mood. We've all felt shattered from time to time and know how easy it is to put off workouts and choose a cup of tea and a biscuit as a quick pick-me-up instead.

Sleep deprivation causes our bodies to release an excess of a 'hunger hormone' called ghrelin: so we naturally can't manage our appetites as we should and the temptation is to reach out for sugar-rich snacks for a quick energy fix. Leptin is the hormone that tells our brains that we're satisfied and can stop eating, but we produce far less of this when we are tired. With these hormones working against you, and not with you, losing body fat and keeping it off for ever are so much harder. I believe that our ability to transform our bodies is largely to do with hormones, and not simply willpower. Once you get your body working with you, you provide yourself with the best possible chance of success.

Our clients who regularly sleep for seven hours a night can lose significantly more body fat than those who are sleep-deprived; the difference is staggering. We often see a dramatic uplift in fat loss on post-natal women once the newborns start sleeping through the night – and I've personally experienced that acceleration, when each of my daughters learned what 'sleeping like a baby' actually meant.

Simply put, the better you feel, the more likely you are to train effectively and to eat intelligently and beautifully. There is a very simple system and you need to practise, practise, practise it. It does take some discipline to tear yourself away from a box set, but as soon as you get the habit, you'll love it.

★ **First, work out what time** you need to get up in the morning, so that you have a relaxed start to the day, and time to prepare breakfast and do your workout, if that's when you're going to create the habit.

★ **Work back seven hours** plus an extra 30 minutes: this is your bedtime.

★ **Practise a strict 'screen curfew'** 90 minutes before bed. Screen-light stimulates your brain and prevents you feeling sleepy and – whether it's a mobile, TV or laptop – it's a time-drain and you need to create more time, not less. Record your absolute favourite TV shows and enjoy them before your screen curfew or at the weekend. Set your alarm and, if it is on your phone, put it away in a drawer. It must be out of sight.

★ **Work back 60 minutes** from your bedtime: this is the ideal time to have a warm bath, with four to six drops of essential lavender oil and a half-cup of Epsom salts (unless you have sensitive skin). The magnesium in the Epsom salts will help your muscles relax, and the lavender will have a restful, sedative effect. Plus, as your body cools down from the bath, you will begin to feel very sleepy – which should coincide perfectly with your bedtime.

★ **Ensure that the hour before bed** remains calm and relaxed. Dim the lights and treat yourself to a scented candle and pillow spray. Enjoy classical or soothing music and make sure that your bedroom is neither too cold nor too warm.

★ **Make your bed as gorgeous as can be** – invest in Egyptian cotton or linen sheets, a mattress topper or a silk-filled duvet to regulate your body temperature.

★ **Hop into bed in the most delicious sleepwear** you can afford, and read a real paper book in bed until your eyes wobble, and then you have the ingredients for the most wonderful night's sleep.

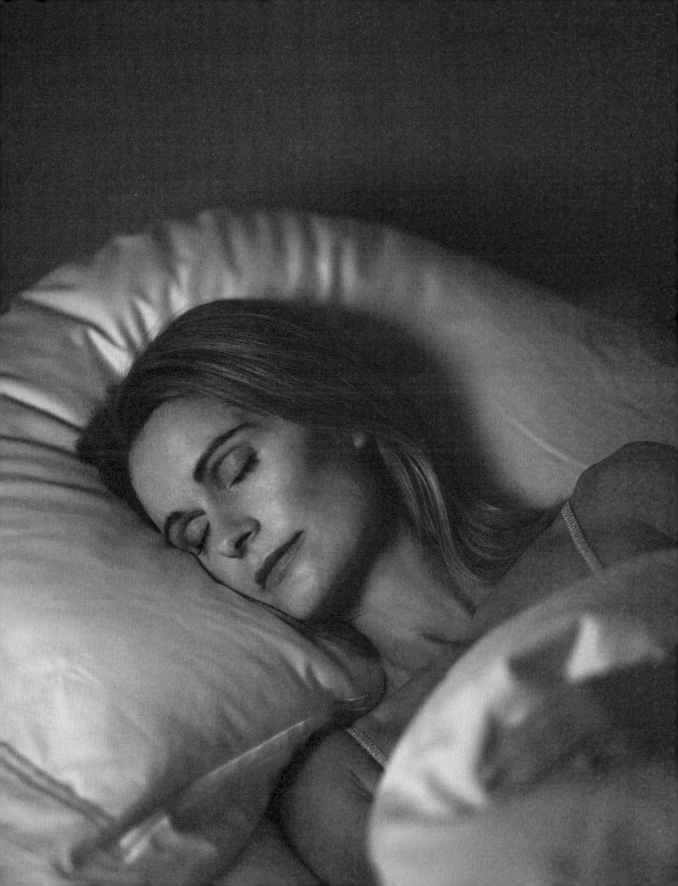

Eliminate Stress

You're going to tackle stress head-on and feel calm and happy.

I'd have been the first to skip this section a decade ago and hum 'Yadee Yadee Yadah', until I saw at first hand how dramatically stress can slow down fat loss. As I began to look after more and more very high-profile clients – CEOs of FTSE 100 companies, politicians and entrepreneurs who lived on a plane and were under constant pressure – the stress issue became something I just couldn't ignore as an afterthought on our programmes.

Stress leads to a long list of health issues, which will reduce the quality of your life: high blood pressure, heart problems, depression and even immune deficiencies. Not to mention the fact that it ruins the ride of your wonderful life. We help each client tackle stress, and the results are significantly stronger across the board – whether the client is a president or a pastry chef. Because regardless of how much pressure there is on you, and the significance of it (a deal worth £8 billion, or 400 cupcakes rising to perfection), to the individual in question, stress is just stress.

When you're really stressed, there's an urge to do something…anything. And it's usually something easy and comforting, like eating or drinking. It's because your high levels of the stress hormone cortisol are tempting you to eat high-carbohydrate food and sugars; and, once you give in to that, you learn the habit, because it's comforting – it works. The next time you're stressed, you do the same, as your brain has learned that this is what you do: it's your behavioural response.

So we are going to break the habit. First, by dramatically reducing your stress so that cortisol doesn't push you in the direction of sugar. And second, by channelling this impulse into something that is good for you, that will actually reduce your stress *and* your bottom size; and, once you've broken the cycle, your brain will know this to be your New Normal – it's just what you do now.

If you want to avoid overeating carbohydrates, you have to do so on purpose. When you wake up, you can't simply wait to see what kind of willpower you have that day – you have to decide to get your hormones working with you, to lend you a hand. And part of that is getting stress under control. All this stressing is working against making you leaner or, as I call it, 'leaning you out'.

I think of stress as falling into four categories: Lion Stroking, Shark Attacks, Scorpion Bites and Mossie Bites.

Lion Stroking

Stroking a lion is *good* stress. It's what gets you out of bed in the morning, excites you and makes you feel alive. Lion Stroking is when you lean into life, take a risk and 'feel the fear, but do it anyway'. It's when you walk onstage to speak to a room of 400 people and you decide to go note-free. It's the feeling you have when you're writing a book and are terrified that only your mother will buy it. It's handing the guy at baggage reclaim your phone number and hoping he doesn't laugh at you. Without it, life would be tediously boring and we'd all still be living in caves. I believe you have to stroke lions to live your best life.

Shark Attacks

Shark Attacks are bad, but thankfully rare. Such attacks come out of nowhere and leave you struggling for months. You either bring it on yourself by swimming in dangerous waters or it's an extraordinarily unfortunate and painful part of life's rich tapestry.

Shark Attacks are when your live-in boyfriend sleeps with your very best friend; you find out that someone you love is knocking on the Pearly Gates; or you're facing the prospect of losing your home. Shark Attacks are terrifying and you can hardly eat or sleep, but you always survive them. And if you feel you haven't survived yet, then the healing process just hasn't finished – but it always will heal. You can't always prevent a Shark Attack, but you can control how you react to them.

Scorpion Bites

Scorpion Bites are bad news and you may carry around the stress for days, weeks or months. It's when you've fallen out with your sister; you've lost 20 per cent of your savings on a really bad investment; or have been gazumped on your dream home. You always survive Scorpion Bites, but it does take time to get over them. Unless you pull the sting out, they hang over you like a black cloud, making each Scorpion Bite somehow much more irritating and harder to deal with.

Mossie Bites

Mossie Bites are bloody irritating. It's when you drop buttered toast on your silk blouse ten minutes before

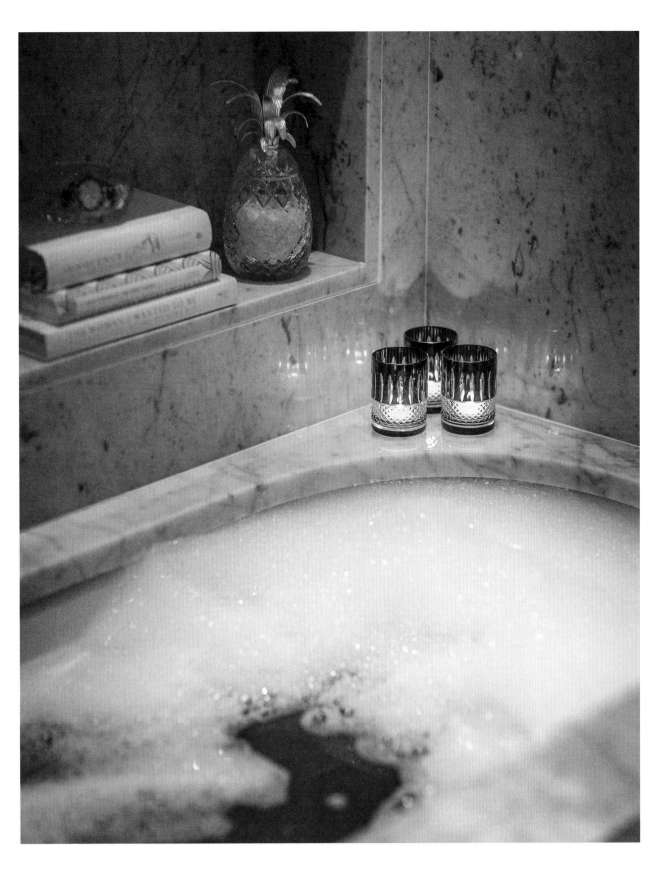

work; when you look at your diary on a Sunday night and there's not even time to go to the loo. It's when you've taken on too much and you have to call someone and let them down, or when your daughter spills nail varnish on your brand-new carpet. Your heart races, you're snappy and feel like you need a Valium smoothie. Some days you can be covered in Mossie Bites and nothing will ruin your mood, and on others just one bite can send you into a spin, if your limbs are also covered in Scorpion Bites.

Unlike Shark Attacks, which give you that temporary loss of appetite, the chronic, constant stress of Scorpion Bites and Mossie Bites cause weight gain.

How Stress Causes Weight Gain

A common perception is that stress causes weight loss. We probably all know of someone who's dropped 1 stone after a massive shark attack. Acute anxiety will temporarily kill your appetite, and as adrenalin soars through your body, you can drop weight fast – often taking precious muscle mass with it. So while we might console our friend with 'every cloud has a silver lining', the effect is actually negative. You lose muscle and therefore lower your metabolism.

Here's why: the chronic stress of Scorpion and Mossie Bites increases your appetite. You physically increase your body's desire for carbohydrates, which ultimately leads to detrimental habits falling into place, if the stress is constant. The hormones push you into the habit of finding comfort in food, whilst the stresses engulf your motivation, enthusiasm and optimism.

It's all to do with our neuroendocrine system. This is the 'brain-to-body' pathway that was essential for our survival in Paleolithic times, and we needed this 'fight or flight' messaging in order to survive being chased by an 8ft bear, which back then was probably no more than a Scorpion Bite. Sadly, this body system is still very finely tuned, even though today we really only need it if we're trapped in a lift. However, it's activated *whenever* you feel threatened or stressed – even if it's just a little Mossie Bite.

Our bodies quickly release adrenalin (which is that warm wave of instant energy that quickly gets your arse into gear) with a dose of cortisol and corticotropin-releasing hormone (CRH). The adrenalin and CRH temporarily lower your appetite, but this is fleeting. The cortisol hangs about; its role is to replenish the body long after the stress has passed (regardless of the severity of the bite). It drives you to eat more, and to store body fat in the visceral area – deep within your tummy and around your organs, which puts you at risk of a shopping list of diseases and may be why you can never quite lean out around the tummy.

Your body wants to transport blood sugars to your muscles and, to move the sugar from your blood to wherever it's needed, your body has to release insulin (the fat-storage hormone), as it's the hormone that opens the door to the cells and lets the sugar in. And high sugar and insulin levels mean one thing – fat gain.

So whilst you're blaming yourself for tucking into a bagel, it's actually a physical, biological human urge. That's not to say you can let yourself off the hook, blame your hormones and slather your bagel in jam – but you need to recognize that it's the hormones setting the stage for a carbohydrate blowout. And if you know how to control and stabilize your hormones through the lifestyle changes of improving sleep (see page 38) and reducing your stress, then you set yourself up for success. It's too easy to blame stress for a slower result – eating in response to stress is encouraged by brain chemistry, but it is also a habit we can unravel – but you need to face the stress head-on.

Life is constantly throwing challenges at us, but it's about taking control of everything that comes your way, knowing that you are doing the next right thing and taking action. When you tackle procrastination, you will feel free, but it requires constant tending. I have a little mantra of 'Do it Now' – and I simply deal with anything that's depleting my mood, there and then. The only way to feel free is to do the work, and it's so much easier to take the direct route. You're going to have to do it, so it might as well be now.

How to Dramatically Reduce Stress

Here's what I recommend to turn down the dial on *all* types of stress. These strategies are part of the Louise Parker Method and they will have a profound impact on reducing all the varieties of stress in your life.

Actively beat stress through what you eat

You're going to create a celebration around every meal and snack.

Eating five mini-meals a day, with a balance of macronutrients (rather than carb-heavy food or three big meals a day), will keep those blood-sugar levels steady, preventing insulin production and energy spikes – this is going to reduce your cortisol levels and control your body-fat levels (especially around the midriff) and your appetite. Your new style of eating, which is higher in fibre and protein, will control blood-sugar levels and prevent hunger.

You'll cut out alcohol during the Transform Phase (and significantly reduce it in the Lifestyle Plan), which sends insulin and cortisol levels soaring towards fat gain. You're going to balance your caffeinated drinks, as an excess can also cause cortisol to rise. You're going to eat an abundantly nutritious diet, ensuring that you get plenty of B-complex vitamins, Vitamin C, calcium and magnesium – all of which are needed to balance cortisol and burn fat, and which can be depleted by stress. You'll regularly eat foods that are rich in the mood regulator serotonin in the array of whole foods in every recipe. Everything in beautiful balance will result in happy, healthy hormones.

Actively beat stress through moving

You're going to exercise every day, no matter what.

Exercise is the best stress-buster. I've never, ever gone for a workout after a horrendous day and not come back feeling infinitely better. Working out at a challenging (but not brutal) level has an astonishing effect on your stress levels, both in the short and long term. Exercise reduces the stress hormone, cortisol (unless it's extreme exercise, which you won't be doing), and increases the happy, feel-good hormones that instantly improve your mood.

Endorphins: These are natural chemicals that interact with your brain and which, when released through exercise, produce a 'high' similar to that of opiates – making you feel really positive, increasing pleasure and reducing pain in the body. They're also released when you feel excited, experience love, eat spicy food and have great sex. I hope you'll experience all these wonders over the coming weeks.

Serotonin: Exercising increases the level of tryptophan in the brain, causing the amino acid that is used to produce serotonin, which is the 'happy hormone'. A deficiency or difficulty in the uptake of serotonin will lead to depression. Serotonin is also stimulated by sunlight and diet – both of which you will be nailing, as we aim to get you working out gym-free and outdoors much more often.

Dopamine: This is a 'feel-good' and motivation neurohormone. It's the chemical that enables pleasure in the brain, and is released when you do many parts of my Method (exercise, reaching goals, having sex) and some you will not do (taking drugs).

Every time you tick off a workout on the Louise Parker Method, or another small accomplishment – a good night's sleep, dealing with a nagging worry, preparing your meals for the following day, anything that consistently moves you towards your goal – you will get a little hit of dopamine. And dopamine feels good, so it's going to motivate you to keep working towards your goal and the little hit of happiness that comes with it. The level of dopamine in your body actually helps to determine how consistent you are at achieving your goals.

As brain chemistry is understood more and more, it's being shown that consistent (there's that word again) exercise helps prepare pathways in the brain, so that we can deal with all stress and anxiety in a much more positive way, not just at the moment when we have finished the workout – but around the clock and habitually. So whilst your workout will quickly eradicate stress through the release of all these feel-good hormones, when you really make a habit change to work out every day, you'll get this longer-term benefit of being able to handle stress in a much calmer and healthier way – which is truly incredible.

Practise daily pleasures

You're going to punctuate your day with a handful of pleasures.

What is happiness to you? Think about the pleasures in your day-to-day life and avoid taking your mind to the future, money or material things. Focus on people, pleasures and pastimes.

I'm the first to confess that I'm more Joan Collins than Dalai Lama, and one of my best friends calls me 'WantyWanty'. There isn't an Amish bone in my body and I truly love luxury in any form: beautiful fabrics, art, hardback books, fabulous clothes, Manolo Blahniks, buttery leather handbags and luxury holidays. I love quality, detail and beauty. I'm not apologetic about this, either – I think it's no bad thing, as long as I do good work for it and know in my heart what truly matters.

It's tempting for me to say that happiness is a soft grey Birkin and a week at Sandy Lane – and, don't get me wrong, this would make me squeal – but it is short-lived: holidays end, and there's *always* another handbag.

So whilst aspiring for places and things isn't bad, you have to truly get pleasure from living in your present, wherever you are, whatever your situation. It's the pleasures that punctuate our every day that truly make us happy. It's utterly pointless living a life that is 95 per cent painful, tedious and utterly stressful, just so that you can strive for 5 per cent of your precious time on a luxury holiday.

For a moment, forget the big gestures – the things your mind goes to when you think, 'If only I had that, I'd be happy.' Think about the parts of your day, your life, *today*, that give you the greatest pleasure. The moments that warm you from the inside. It's probably the simple things: sitting for a moment on your own with a coffee with perfect, thick froth; cuddling under a blanket with your child on your chest, feeling the rhythm of his or her breath; or making love to your husband (ideally *not* someone else's), slowly and sleepily.

Make a list of four things in your everyday life that bring you great pleasure. It's not many, and it's all you need to sprinkle your day with 'Aaaahs'. They must be simple and they can't cost more than a fiver (allowing for a good cappuccino). I want to force you to think about it, ink it and ensure you make time to punctuate your day with these simple pleasures.

These little moments will release dopamine, and they're going to tackle stress by the balls. It's hard to believe that stroking the dog for five minutes will improve your weight loss – but now that you can see the link, it really will. My Method is about living your *best* life, in your best body.

You are in control of your lifestyle. If you don't like it, change it

Brain napping

You're going to 'brain-nap' for 20 minutes a day.

What I am talking about here is actually quieting the mind for 20 minutes, switching off totally and giving it a nap. You can't do this online, watching *Scandal* or liking avocado on toast on Instagram. This is total quiet time – just you and nothing else, not even your thoughts.

Your body and mind will *thrive* if you treat them to a 20-minute 'brain-nap' each day. They'll awaken alert, ready to conquer anything, constructive and creative. I *know* this seems an impossible feat at times, and if all you can manage to begin with is five minutes, do that and build it up: each week add another five minutes, until in Week Four of Transform you're 'brain-napping' for 20 minutes a day.

You can 'brain-nap' in many ways – gardening, walking the dog, zoning out in the bath or simply lying on your bed with a sleep-mask on. Meditation is the most profoundly effective way of 'brain-napping' and, if you already meditate, fantastic – put it back in your schedule. I have to be honest: I've tried numerous times to learn traditional meditation, using guided chanting and sitting in the pose, fingers together, and it hasn't worked for me – yet. It's on my to-do list, along with yoga and Italian; and that's okay: it's good to have things to keep in my Innovation Box. But I meditate in my own way, and if the 'Om Namah Shivaya' variety doesn't work for you, then you need to find you own style.

Whenever that feeling of stress stirs in your belly, it's time to 'brain-nap'. If the office is stressful, escape to a window and stare out of it for a few minutes. If you've three children tugging at you, sit in the bathroom, shut your eyes and just think about nothing for as long as it's safe to leave them unattended. It's not going to happen by accident – you need to pop in a 'brain-nap' whenever you feel you need it. Even if your day has been calm, slot in your 'brain-nap' and build up reserves for a stormier day.

Walking to my office is my 'brain-napping'. It's a 20-minute brisk walk, through Battersea Park, over Chelsea Bridge, Pimlico Green and to my clinic in Belgravia. It's part of my 'active rest' and always relaxes me and kicks the day off on a strong footing.

I zone out and think about nothing. When my mind races and my to-do list takes over my brain, I bring myself back to exactly where I am – the smell of the rain in Battersea Park; how the cold air feels on my face; each muscle in my body working; the flow of the River Thames; the lights

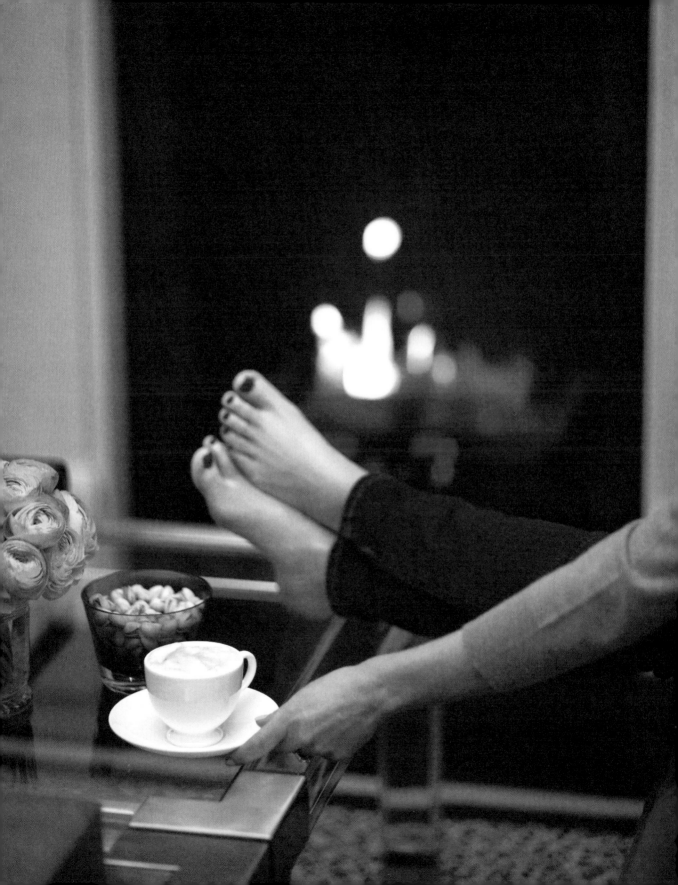

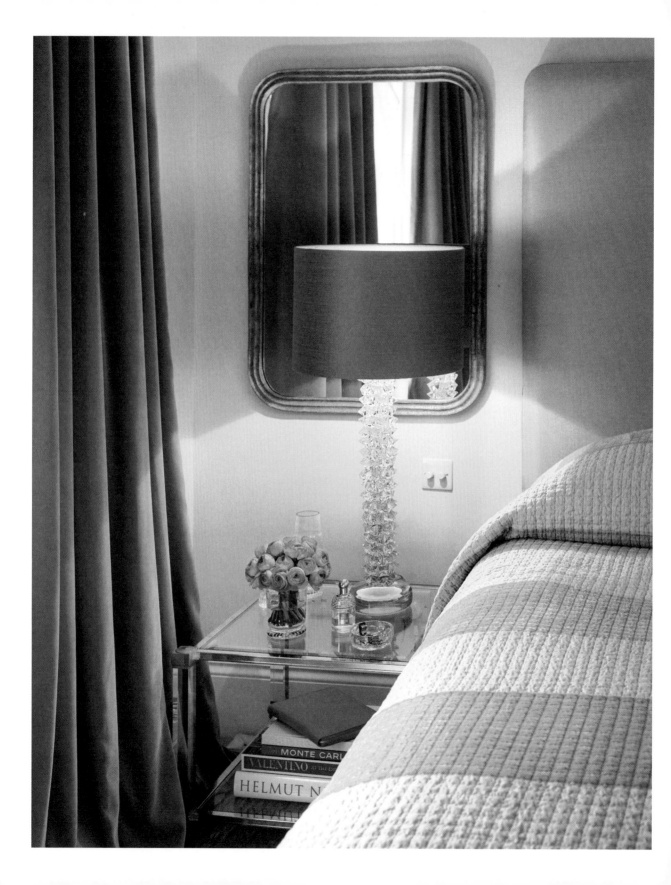

on Albert Bridge at night, twinkling at me and reminding me I am almost home. I keep pulling my mind back to the present, to the moment. I make sure I'm warm and comfortable and I never listen to music. I block out the noise of the traffic, creating a little soundproof bubble around me, where nothing can disturb me. It's just what I do, and I love it. It's become my daily meditation.

When you consistently 'brain-nap', you deal with stress phenomenally better. You take control of your mind, allowing it to rest, zone out and recuperate. And from that stillness and calm, the stresses you return to seem to shrink in significance. It works.

Debris detox

You're going to identify what's eating at you, ink it and deal with it.

Clearing out the physical debris (your fabulous declutter at home) and the mental debris that may be eating away at you, will set you free. And I want you to be 'fit, happy and free'.

You need to eliminate the real causes of your stress, and the only way to do that is to identify them, write them down, plan an attack and crack on with it. Don't ignore or put off a solution to anything that is compromising your happiness. Anything that you've put to the back of your mind for now is still in your mind. To tick it off your mental list of worries, the only way through it is *straight* through it.

What I have discovered is, if you don't learn a lesson you're meant to, or address whatever's eating at you or make a decision that's pending, it keeps coming back at you, a little stronger every time – until you face it, deal with it, make a decision and move on.

Let it go

You're going to let go completely.

Given that I've a toddler with a *Frozen* obsession, I am thankfully reminded in song of this little adage on a daily basis – and my daughter CoCo does seem to burst into delightful song whenever I am festering upon something I shouldn't. Once you have dealt with all the bites and burdens weighing you down, truly 'Let It Go'. Letting go is really just a decision. You can decide to keep gossiping about it, moaning about it, allowing it to tread water in your mind – or, every time it pops into your head, literally tell it where to go. You've made a decision, dealt with it: now let it be. Every time you allow the bite to linger in your mind, you're allowing yourself to be nibbled at again,

Fit, happy and free

and all these nibbles will stress you out. Letting go is a habit, and a habit of highly happy and successful people – so keep practising until it becomes a part of who you are.

Change your language

You're going to talk positively about the change you are making.

The way you think about and vocalize your worries dictates the power they have over you. Keep adding your bites to an ongoing list, and keep dealing with them. Be very careful of the language that you use around your friends and family as you talk about what's going on in your life. If you enter into competitive stress or tiredness syndrome with your friends, it's going to end up dragging you down, not up.

I'm not saying you should behave like a Stepford Wife and not share honestly – but try to put a positive spin on it, and avoid 'stinking thinking' (see page 31). For a whole week try not to say that you are tired or stressed, and see the difference it has on your mood. Remember not to say to yourself, or anyone else, that you are 'on a diet' – which you are not. 'I'm making some changes I should have made long ago' will be totally empowering and won't invite opinions that you haven't asked for.

Design your perfect day

You're going to create your ideal day.

Remember that you are in control of your lifestyle. If you don't like it, change it. It may not happen overnight, but you can design your lifestyle to be whatever you want it to be. Don't be afraid to sit down and actually write out what your ideal lifestyle would be – and then think about what steps you can take to achieve it. Visualize it, ink it and make a plan. Think about what's important to you – what you'd fill your time with, what work you'd do – and basically design 'A Day in the Life' of your alter ego.

It's an exercise I do at the start of each school term – I design my daily routine, to keep things interesting and to force me to look at my lifestyle and make sure I'm punctuating my day with things that ensure I'm productive, happy and fulfilled. You define your life's story and your body's health by the daily decisions and habits you make. You are in the driving seat.

Keep careful company

You're going to surround yourself with cheerleaders.

Transformation and building a healthy new lifestyle require support from those around you. One of the reasons our success rate is so extraordinary with the Louise Parker Method is that our clients are fully supported and have someone to advise, motivate and encourage them throughout their journey. I think that, more than being accountable to someone else, it's about being accountable to *yourself* – and with each week that you tick off you get a buzz that propels you forward.

Make sure that you surround yourself with positive people. Make a list of Uppers and Downers, and brutally divide all the people in your life into these two camps. I realize it sounds brutal, but it's about recognizing who encourages you, bringing positivity, inspiration and fun into your life. Just be aware of who they are, and think about which group you spend most of your time with. If you're spending time with judgemental, critical people who don't back your dreams, you risk not realizing your potential. Surround yourself with what you perceive as success – whether that's empathy, good values, entrepreneurism, joie de vivre or loyalty.

Be acutely aware that there will be people in your life who don't want you to succeed. They may envy your enthusiasm, drive and determination and, ultimately, your results. Those around you often don't want you to change…and my Method *will* change you. Just keep your wits about you and recognize who is trying to sabotage you with comments like 'Oh, don't be so boring – you can take one weekend off' or 'Don't lose too much weight –

it's not a good look at our age'. Learn to block out these opinions and let them blow right over you. Most of the time it's their issues that are the problem and not yours, so learn to let negative and uninvited opinions wash over you. Remember that your job is to stay in the inner circle, even when someone tries to tempt you or push you out.

Form a positive tribe

You're going to create a support group.

Surround yourself with a tribe of people who share your goals. It will have the most astonishing effect on your results. Be brave and be the first one to pick up the phone, to see if they'll join you.

Ideally there should be at least four of you in each group. Try to stretch your tribe beyond three, so that there's always a good turnout of enthusiasm and optimism on any given day.

Ask your friends, colleagues and neighbours to join in, set a date on which you'll all start and work out how you'll support each other. Discuss what's going to work for you all: perhaps it's a Skype call, if you're dotted all over the world, or an hour in your favourite coffee shop after the school run. Whatever you decide, make sure the time and day are absolutely set in stone, and do not move them, no matter what. Put the date in your diary and commit to it. This is why it's good to have up to eight of you – it will help you stick to the time. Do not move it for one person; they'll just have to slot in the following week. By moving the date, you'd belittle the value you place on it, so give it the commitment it deserves.

Once you've completed the programme and switched to the after-party, keep the support going, as you may have friends who are still in the Transform Phase, and it will really help you to motivate other people as you consolidate the habits into your New Normal. Giving it back and passing it on will strengthen you.

Find support that is kind, caring and committed

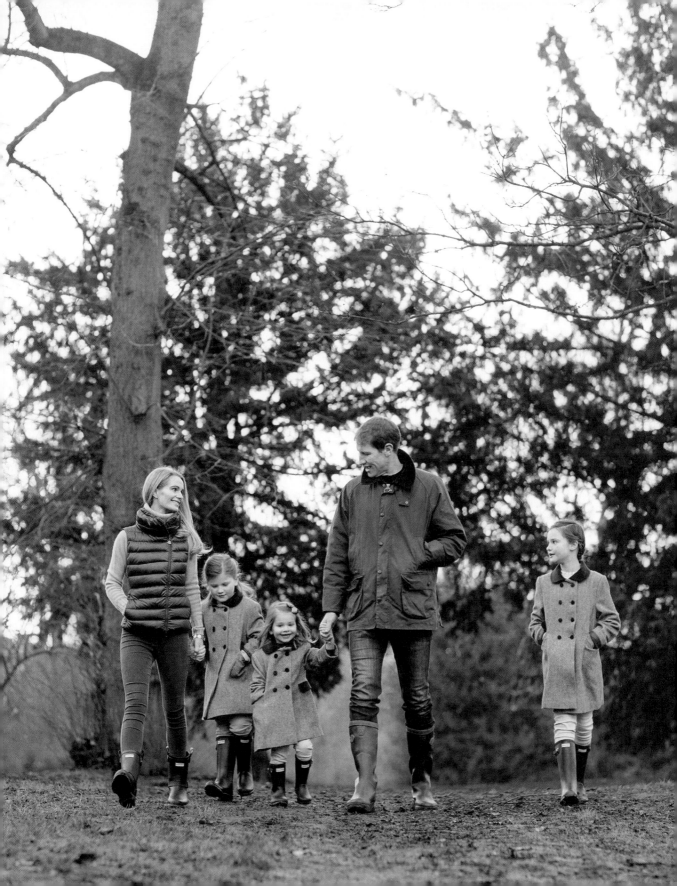

3

★ Eat 3 meals and 2 snacks per day. You've a choice of 80 recipes, each super-simple and quick to prepare

★ Start your day with 'Lemonize' and stay well hydrated throughout

EAT BEAUTIFULLY

There are five principles to my nutritional method that I'd like you to understand before you begin. Understanding the concept of the Food Plan (please never call it a diet) makes it easier for you to fully commit to your new style of eating. The core principles (see page 54) are super-simple to put into practice and, because you'll understand the purpose of each point, you'll be assured that your new style of eating makes total sense – and there'll be no going back.

I'm interested in two things on the programme: getting you the best possible fat-burning results, in a way that's so sustainable that the style of eating is going to become a habit. Remember that motivation is temporary, but habits last a lifetime.

Because I want to pull extraordinary results out of the bag, I layer all the principles that drive the best fat loss into one plan – carefully weaving them together so that every trick of the trade is condensed into my Method. I'll explain each principle in the following section and it's important

that you take each one on board, so that eventually you'll be directing your own meals each day, like second nature.

The principles of the plan are precise, but they do allow for the most beautiful variety and range of meals – the possibilities are literally endless. Once you absorb the approach, you'll be throwing together combinations and relying less on my recipes. I can literally look at any recipe and adapt it to suit my Method, and you'll soon learn how to do this, too.

Remember: this is not a diet, but a style of eating that will form the foundation of the way you eat for ever. I want you to fully embrace it and put love and effort into each and every meal and snack. If you approach it like a 'diet' and eat cold chicken and iceberg lettuce for lunch, you're sabotaging your chances of success. You're telling yourself that it's miserable and setting yourself up to fail. No meal or snack should feel depressing and, if it does, you're just not doing it right.

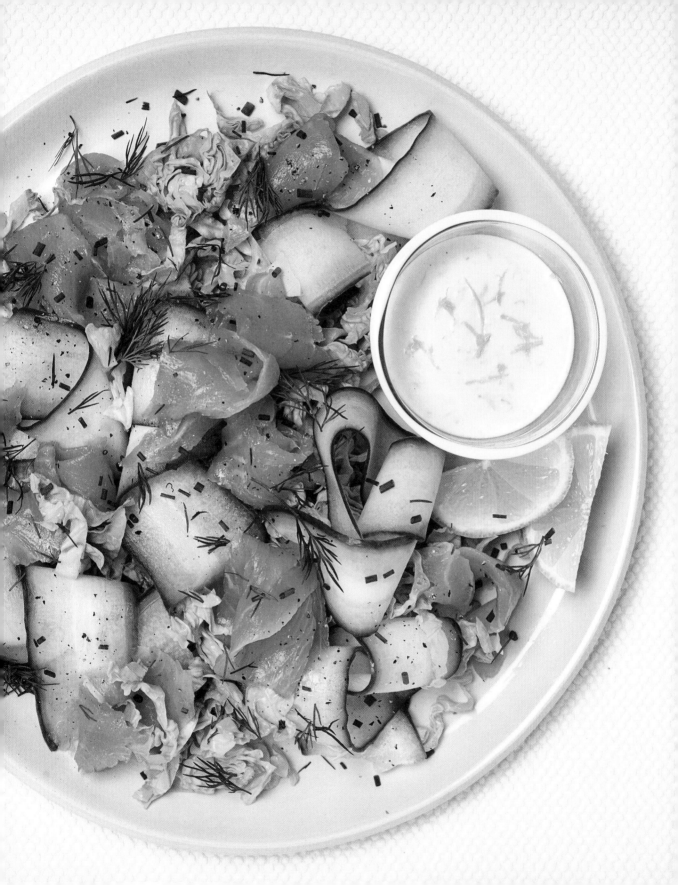

Most people have a repertoire of about 20 recipes that form the basis of what they eat much of the time – either when cooking at home or when eating out in a restaurant. If my husband cooks dinner, I have a good idea that it'll be one of about 20 possibilities, and I can pretty much guess what he'll go for on a restaurant menu. He's not a particularly tedious man – I think it's just what we all do.

Try to think of this plan as simply re-jigging your list of foundation recipes. What will happen is that you'll find new favourites to upgrade the options you've been cooking for years. It's so easy to get stuck in the rut of eating the same midweek meals because it's become a habit. New, beautifully delicious meals are now going to become a habit for you. You'll continually try new dishes and refresh your favourites, particularly when the seasons change and your body craves either comforting food or lighter summer dishes.

Once you reach your goal, we're slowly going to reintroduce the celebratory foods that you feel are 'worth it', so that you can sit down in your favourite restaurant and order whatever jumps out at you. You'll pop over to friends for dinner and happily eat whatever you're given, because no food is 'naughty' or 'a sin' – especially when you're eating it in perfect balance with the most nutritious and healthy foundations.

With my Method you don't need a 'maintenance' plan, as you'll be happily in the habit of eating deliciously lean, clean meals that you love most of the time. You'll be eating this way roughly 80 per cent of the time, allowing you to eat and drink whatever pleases you roughly 20 per cent of the time. Anything you've missed

horribly (like ice-cream on Sundays or Saturday-morning croissants) you can simply ease back into your style of eating in balance. Please don't confuse this with 'dieting' and 'cheat days', because neither do I want you horribly overeating 20 per cent of the time. And please never call a cake a treat – it's not – it's just cake.

Your appetite and tastes will change as your figure does, so you'll be surprised by what you actually want to eat with abandon, when the majority of your meals are clean and healthy. There's a huge difference between enjoying a steak and French fries with a couple of glasses of claret and polishing off a packet of Hobnobs in front of the TV. You're going to eat beautifully, mindfully and with celebration all of the time – whether it's a leaner or a more celebratory meal (never a 'cheat meal').

During the Transform Phase you're going to follow the nutrition plan 100 per cent of the time. This isn't because I'm a gym-mistress, but because the direct route is the easy route, and 'treating yourself' to a day when you ruin four days' effort isn't really a treat at all. It's sabotage and this habit will always keep you at arm's length from true success – so you need to break the cycle. Stopping and restarting is a boring habit in itself and means the results take infinitely longer.

You are aiming for something special in terms of results, and so you can't put in average effort. Play close attention to all the suggestions, and day-by-day you'll realize that you're just getting on with it, without even thinking about it. The thought, concentration and planning are all simply temporary measures until the habit-change kicks in – which it will for you, as it does for everyone.

Avoid Becoming Organically Overweight

There are so many great healthy-eating books on the bestseller list at the moment that celebrate whole food that is beautiful, virtuous and wonderfully nutritious. But it's important not to confuse this with weight loss. There is a big difference between clean eating and lean eating.

We've seen a phenomenal rise of clients at Louise Parker who have been following 'clean' recipes and feel really confused as to why they've put on significant weight. Keep your wits about you – and know that a coconut yogurt with 2 cups of granola, agave nectar and cocoa nibs is gorgeous and nutritious, but is just as laden with sugars as a chocolate cake may be. In many cases, even more so.

It's one thing to know that you're overweight because you're on first-name terms with the pizza delivery man,

but another to be doing what you think is 'healthy', but is in fact laden with hidden calories and sugars – it's what we call 'organically overweight'. We are bombarded with organic, seasonal, wholefood porn – and whilst I'm not for a minute saying this isn't a good thing, it can mislead people into a style of eating whereby they think calories don't matter and are then understandably disheartened when they don't lose weight.

Instagram is awash with skinny girls posting images of coconut porridge with caramelized prunes and agave nectar. Delicious – yes; organic – yes; whole food – yes; nutritious – yes. But calorie-wise it's a match for my mother's sticky-toffee pudding and best not consumed for breakfast daily, if your goal is to look like the girl in the picture. What you can't see is that perhaps she doesn't eat it, or that she works as a personal trainer for eight hours a day.

Paleo and keto diets are other popular trends which, in my opinion, are unsustainable and just not healthy for mind or body. Whilst I'm an advocate of eating protein at every meal, my focus is on balance. It's a foundation principle of my food plan that we pay very close attention to portion sizes and what the overall balance is. A Paleo fan with a daily CrossFit habit may be able to get away with snacking on raw cocoa and nut-balls between meals, but if you're in a sedentary job and an occasional light exerciser, you can't burn off the energy – no matter how pure the ingredients are. Whilst eating a raw food bar of cashew nuts, cocoa and honey may be nutritious, if you don't have the energy requirements of an athlete, your body will assimilate the sugars and fats and, as they hit your bloodstream, you will lay down fat, just as you would have done if you'd eaten a KitKat Chunky.

The trick is to eat whole, real, seasonal, nutritious food. Eating whole food is essentially a wise move, but the sugar and calorie content has to be balanced in a way that stabilizes your blood-sugar levels and creates a gentle calorific deficit, whilst boosting you with nutrients, to create an impressive and sustainable fat loss. Just don't forget your common sense. If you're eating three boiled eggs between meetings, it's neither sustainable, wise or normal.

How to Eat with Celebration & Beauty

The preparation of your meals is almost as important as the meals themselves. We want to encourage you to practise 'eating with ceremony' and there are a few tricks you can learn to start eating beautifully.

Think how you would feel if you were on CCTV? Would you be ashamed to be seen eating as you do? If so, don't do it to yourself, because how you feel about yourself is far more important than what others think about you. Apply the 'Instagram test' and feel proud of the effort and self-care you put into everything you prepare. The positivity it infuses you with is astounding and boosts your motivation overall.

★ **Buy the very best ingredients** you can afford, and store, prepare and arrange your food as beautifully as you can.

★ **Sit at a table to eat and lay it beautifully**, even if you are eating alone. It needn't take more than a minute, once you're in the habit, and you'll instantly enjoy your meals so much more. Invest in the most gorgeous plates, cutlery, napkins and place mats that you can, little by little. It needn't cost a fortune but should make you happy.

★ **Make a commitment to certain meals** of the week being with all the family or special friends and create the time so that you can relax, enjoy the conversation and make a special effort with the meal. It can be done, if you prioritize it.

★ **Never eat standing up. Ever.** You'll drop a dress size alone by adopting this habit. Be mindful of what your body really wants to eat, prepare it well and always, always eat sitting down.

★ **Always eat with screens off**. By not eating in front of a box set or whilst checking your email, your brain will register that you've consciously eaten a beautiful meal. Your email, work and life can always wait 20 minutes. Occasionally enjoy a TV supper, but lay a tray beautifully.

★ **Think ahead and prepare your 'on-the-go' snacks** as if you were doing so for your best friend. A little pot of salted pecan nuts, with a ziplock bag of fresh cherries in your bag, makes your snacks so much nicer than grabbing something last-minute from a petrol station and eating in the car. You have to prepare to make snacking a pleasure – it won't just accidentally happen.

CORE PRINCIPLES

1
LOVE FLAVOUR
You're going to cook with flavour, using ingredients that are bursting with freshness, and discover taste combinations that are simple and delicious.

2
CALORIES DO MATTER
Creating a sensible calorific deficit burns through fat storage, doesn't sabotage precious muscle mass and allows you ample calories to sustain your energy levels and workouts, whilst eating a highly nutritious diet.

3
EAT THREE MEALS AND TWO SNACKS PER DAY
Precisely balancing your meals throughout the day stabilizes blood-sugar levels, appetite, mood and hormones, enabling optimum fat-burning, and making it easy to stick to my Method long-term.

4
ALWAYS BALANCE YOUR FOOD GROUPS
Combining a little of each macronutrient (protein, fat, carbohydrate) at each meal supports the balancing of blood-sugar levels and hormones. This helps to regulate your mood and appetite so that you feel good.

5
SIP, SIP, SIP
Optimum hydration aids the fat burning process and you'll build the habit of drinking more every day. You'll start each day with my Lemonize drink to rehydrate and boost kidney function.

1 LOVE FLAVOUR

You're going to cook with flavour, using foods bursting with freshness, and discover simple taste combinations that are delicious. You'll cook with spices, herbs and condiments and make sure that every single meal and snack is exploding with gorgeous flavour – without resorting to making your own chicken stock, searching for bizarre ingredients that you can't pronounce or spending Sundays doing weekly food prep when all you truly want is fit, fast food.

I toyed with giving you my granola recipe, but to be honest, I only made it a dozen times and now buy a perfectly good version that is available in supermarkets.

We have to think long-term here – and keep referring to the question 'Will I still be doing this in five years' time?' Five years on and three children later, I buy stock cubes and I don't lose any sleep over it. Pick your battles.

Eating beautifully is not about eating tedious chicken salads from the 1980s. You're going to snazz up super-simple recipes – none of them complicated – to make sure that you really feel satisfied and have eaten a lovely meal, and not some form of punishment. My Method makes the science wonderfully simple, and will lean you out once and for all.

2 CALORIES DO MATTER

What you eat, and how much you eat, determines whether you lay down fat reserves, maintain your existing fat levels or burn body fat. If you eat more calories than your body's basal metabolic rate (BMR) and activity levels, then your cells will get more glucose than they need. If your body does not use it up, it is sent to fat storage. Plain and simple. **By the time this pesky fat cell is sitting on your body, it doesn't matter if it's come from organic coconut porridge or sticky-toffee pudding.** So whilst it's become hugely unpopular to talk about calories and simply eat whole, real food, that's only part of the story. Calories absolutely do matter, if you want to get lean and stay lean.

How many calories your own body needs is determined by your BMR, and this is totally driven by how much muscle you have on your body; so the stronger you are, the greater your daily calorific needs are and the more you can get away with eating. This is why I don't believe that anyone has a 'bad metabolism'. You may have less muscle mass, as a result of years of crash dieting stripping a little away with every diet, but you can correct this and it truly doesn't take long. So if you feel that your metabolism isn't great, just get started. We'll protect it as we lean you out, and then increase it as you get stronger and more defined.

Calories, however, are not all equal – their origin really affects your results, and so I pay close attention to where calories come from and in what balance you distribute them throughout your day. An excess of calories from protein is going to have less of a fat-gain impact than an excess of carbohydrate calories, but at the end of the day if you overeat too much of anything, you're going to gain fat.

Just as you can be 'organically overweight' by eating a diet rich in whole, organic, natural food (so prevalent now with new clients that we've sadly had to create a term for it; see page 52), so can you slow down your fat-burning tap if you pay no attention to the portions of your meals on my plan. It'll still work – but the results will be far less impressive.

However, counting calories and points is totally tedious, so I've created the Method in such a way that you won't need to. I've honestly not counted a calorie that I've eaten since 1997 – instead I'm in the habit of measuring and eating perfect portions by sight. And so will you be soon.

All the calculations are done for you, so all you need to do is keep an eye on each portion of protein, fat and carbohydrate that makes up each meal. In the first couple of weeks you'll need to play close attention to the measures I've given you, but you'll soon learn to measure visually what your portions should look like, and your body will get used to eating more delicate portions. It's basically a fortnight of thinking and effort before it becomes a doddle.

My Method is going to pack in as much nutrition as possible into your daily calorific allowance. We're going to feed you a little more than your BMR requires, but not enough calories to fuel your activities, pottering and workouts. Whilst you'll have plenty of energy to perform them, you won't have enough calories to fuel them, so your fat-burning tap will be dripping every day that you are on Transform. Drip-drip-drip…until you reach your ultimate goal. Keep that vision in mind when you're tempted to turn the tap off.

3 EAT THREE MEALS AND TWO SNACKS PER DAY

It is essential to spread the intake of your calories, proteins and carbohydrates evenly throughout the day to stabilize blood-sugar levels and hormones, preserve your muscle mass and maximize fat-burning. By balancing blood-sugar levels, you support healthy hormone function, which dictates how you feel and how efficiently you lose fat. Stable hormone function combined with steady 'slow-release' energy into your blood system throughout the day will ensure the very best appetite control possible, and your body will finally be able to remove excess fat efficiently because there's no longer an excess of sugar in your system.

So whilst calories matter, it's not simply a question of sticking to a certain amount each day. Someone eating the same number of calories on a slimming-group programme will lose far less body fat than someone eating the same amount of calories with my Method. They're also likely to be really hungry and unable to sustain it for long. The 'diet' fails the client but they blame themselves, return and business booms.

The Louise Parker Method focuses on the building blocks of your meals in a specific ratio, to ensure that you are scientifically burning as much body fat as you can, whilst making it extremely easy to stick to. Again, there are two reasons for this: to keep the fat-burning tap dripping steadily; and, crucially, to make sure that you're comfortable, feeling good and not even slightly hungry, so that it doesn't occur to you to step out of the circle.

You may feel 'peckish' for a few days as you adjust to not overeating, but you'll be surprised by how well your appetite is managed when you are eating to my Method. Managing appetite is integral to both short- and long-term weight loss and, as you permanently shift your style of eating, you'll build the blueprint for long-term success.

One of the biggest causes of weight gain is emotional comfort-eating and cravings, which I believe are curable, simply by eating the right foods at the right time. Food is literally a drug that can positively manipulate your appetite – so let's control your cravings, and not let your cravings control you. It's really not about willpower, so let's leave this 'stinking thinking' behind.

To achieve this, we ensure that you eat every few hours, and focus on eating three good meals and snacks a day. You're going to eat breakfast, a mid-morning snack, lunch, a decent afternoon snack and a light dinner in the evening. I'll help you achieve this whether you're at home or on the go, as from now on you're going to stop skipping meals.

This balance of mini-meals spread across the day ensures that you'll have excellent energy levels and helps beat tiredness – essential for an active lifestyle. Quite simply, the better you feel, the more you'll immerse yourself in the good habits of my Method.

4 ALWAYS BALANCE YOUR FOOD GROUPS

All the food groups are included in each meal and snack in the Louise Parker Food Plan. It's important not to eliminate any whole group or make it the enemy, and lean towards a balanced approach that your body's cells and immunity require to stay healthy. So we want to make sure that your body is regularly fed all the main nutrients it needs.

Each macronutrient will work together to do all the things we want: balance blood sugar, regulate hormones, burn fat steadily, provide you with good energy and sustain your precious muscle mass. Here's what you will need to include in every single meal and snack:

Low-GI Carbohydrate

You need carbohydrates in your diet, especially when you are active. However, if you want to burn through fat storage, you need to stick to low-GI (Glycaemic Index) carbohydrate, which is slowly absorbed by the body, balance it with fat, protein and fibre, and eat intelligently the right amount at the right time of day. This macronutrient is the one that will have the greatest effect on your results. You will replace all high-GI carbohydrates, which are quickly absorbed (sugar, potatoes, rice, pasta, fruit juice and dried fruit, to name a few), with abundantly nutritious, low-GI foods (such as wholemeal bread, oat bran and a vast array of delicious fruits and vegetables). The Louise Parker Method is a smart, balanced, lower-carbohydrate approach to eating – not to be confused with a low-carbohydrate diet.

Protein

A nutritionally balanced diet requires adequate protein, especially when you're working out. Proteins are basically the building blocks of your body, and your body relies on protein to repair and maintain itself. Every single cell and fluid in your body (except bile and your wee) contains protein – your muscles, your skin, your glands and your life-giving organs. These cells constantly need repairing and sustaining, and you need protein to do that job.

When you digest a protein food, essential amino acids are absorbed, and you need to eat adequate amounts of protein for optimum health, fat loss and, crucially, muscle preservation. These essential amino acids are best taken throughout the day, rather than in one big sitting, so again, you're going to balance a little bit of protein with every meal. We're going to infuse you with amino acids from highly nutritious meats, fish, dairy products and eggs, and from vegetarian sources such as pulses, beans, nuts, nut butters and soya, to name a few.

The other upside of a sufficient protein intake is that, of all the macronutrients, protein takes the most energy to actually digest: 20–30 per cent of the calories in protein are required to break down the complex chain of amino acids, so of 100 calories of chicken that you eat, your body can only actually use 70–80 of them. Compared to the SDA (specific dynamic action) of 5–10 per cent of carbohydrate and 0–3 per cent of fat, this is a wonderful saving.

Protein, especially when combined with fat, also has a really useful effect on suppressing your appetite, by improving the feeling of fullness that you have at the end of a meal – which is going to be incredibly helpful long-term in preventing you overeating.

Essential Fats

Fat stored on your body can't be burned with absolute efficiency without 'new' fat to lend a hand – in the form of dietary fat. The fats that you eat help break down body fat by activating fat-burning pathways through the liver. Think of a mealtime on my Method as cleaning: you are trying to vacuum up the old fat, but you need a bit of new elbow grease to get the job done. Without it, that fat won't be sucked up.

So the oil on your salad not only helps you access stored body fat, but also increases the absorption of all the vitamins and minerals in your meal. Many essential vitamins (such as Vitamins A, D, E and K) are fat-soluble, and so without fat, your body can't absorb them. These vitamins play an essential role in keeping energy levels high, in maintaining concentration and focus and, most of all, muscle health, which you need for a healthy metabolism. Omega-3 fat increases protein concentration and the size of muscular cells in the body, which will help to stimulate the laying down of muscle – fundamental in our quest for your lean, tight body that is easy to maintain. So the fat-rich foods are going to boost flavour and taste sensational whilst you get stronger and boost your metabolism.

We're going to primarily include sources of fat from unsaturated sources, which are abundant in nutrients, help remove 'bad' cholesterol from the arteries and keep your ticker healthy. Adding avocado, olive oil, seeds, nuts and fish oil to your meals not only packs a punch on taste, but these foods are a little harder to digest and so hang around the digestive system for longer – keeping you feeling fuller for longer and away from browsing the fridge. We won't shy away from a bit of butter either.

Portions *do* matter, because fat is densely calorific. But I have a simple way for you to add just enough to all your meals for fat to do its essential job and make every meal more gorgeous.

Fibre

Whilst fibre has no magical fat-burning properties, it's essential for bowel health and helps you feel full for much longer, by simply filling your tummy and telling your brain it's time to stop eating. There's no energy in fibre, so you can do this without adding extra calories to your diet, too. Fibre passes through you and crucially helps to stabilize blood-sugar levels, so it really supports your fat-loss goals.

High-fibre foods have a much lower impact on blood-sugar levels than low-fibre foods – so an orange won't spike levels of insulin (the fat-storage hormone) in the same way that a glass of fruit juice would, with its many concentrated fruits in one hit, stripped of their precious fibre. It's why I'm not a fan of juicing.

You're going to get your fibre intelligently from various sources: fresh strawberries, raspberries and frozen summer berries being some of my favourites, amongst a vast list of totally delicious fresh (and frozen) fruits and vegetables. Fibre keeps you regular, too, pulling waste products from the body and making it more comfortable to go to the loo – especially when you start to increase the amount of protein in your diet, which can have a temporary constipating effect.

Building Blocks

Every meal is made up of specific amounts of these different building blocks. The easiest way to make sure you're getting the right amount of each is simply to follow the recipes I give you. However, because I want you to build good habits, understanding the building blocks is important because it enables you to change the recipes to suit your taste, lifestyle and the food you have in your fridge on any given day.

What Foods Do I Have to Avoid?

There is so much choice and variety in my nutritional method that the combinations and choices really are endless. However, whilst you're on your programme there are some things you need to cut out: alcohol, sugar (and products that contain it), natural sugar alternatives such as honey and agave nectar, fruit juice, refined carbohydrates (white bread, rice, cereals, couscous, pasta), heavily processed foods, diet products and shop-bought smoothies. You'll generally avoid foods with an 'ose' on the end – like sucrose, dextrose and glucose. You'll be eating some fructose from fruit, and some lactose from milk, in balance.

Don't obsess about the foods you can't have; instead, focus on the delicious foods you can eat and the results you will achieve. Enjoy each recipe and don't be afraid to experiment, as long as you stick to the principles. After six weeks, and once your habits have changed, I guarantee that you won't want to reintroduce many of the things you expected to miss as much as you think you will. Instead, you will begin to crave fresh, whole food – I promise.

5 SIP, SIP, SIP

Water is crucial for circulating nutrients around the body and, when you aren't drinking enough, the systems of elimination don't work as well as they should. So you're going to stay really well hydrated, both for the purposes of your transformation and to enable just about every bodily function to operate at its full potential. Sadly, water doesn't flush fat from the body, but if you're dehydrated, your fat-metabolism efforts will be compromised.

That's no surprise when your body is nearly 60 per cent water and your brilliant brain 75 per cent. Feeling sharp, alert and full of energy is one of your main objectives, so you need to make sure you drink plenty. Don't drink an excessive amount, however, as this isn't good for you either. Your daily water needs are entirely personal and come down to so many factors, but aim for 2.5 litres (4½ pints) a day, to start with (increasing this in hot weather or on days when you train your socks off) and let thirst be your guide. If you get thirsty, you're already dehydrated, so you know you need to increase your water intake the following day by at least ½ litre (18fl oz).

Soluble fibre absorbs water and forms a sort of gel-like substance in your gut, which slows down the absorption of sugars in your bloodstream. And, as you already know, lower blood-sugar levels result in lower insulin levels and in your body storing less fat. It's very common to confuse hunger with thirst, so whenever you get the niggle of hunger, drink a large glass of water and wait for ten minutes.

The most effective way to hydrate is by drinking water (mineral or tap water) evenly throughout the day. Limit caffeinated drinks to three per day, as they can have a dehydrating effect and an excess can disrupt your insulin function. I won't be removing your beloved tea and coffee, however – just regulating the milk, and ensuring that it's all in moderation.

We'll need to get you into the habit of simply drinking more every single day – and I'll teach you some tricks you can use to slot in more liquid. Once you're actually used to drinking more, you'll want more – a bit like sex, and going to the movies.

I drink more caffeine than I probably should, but I always have my last cup of coffee at lunchtime and tea at 3pm. From then on, I stick to water and herbal teas.

DRINKING DOS AND DON'TS

Here's the detail about what you will and won't be drinking when you're in your inner circle:

ESSENTIAL DRINK TO START THE DAY

What? 300ml (10fl oz) of 'Lemonize' – Simply squeeze the juice of ½ fresh lemon into a glass. Mix 150ml (5fl oz) of cold water and 150ml (5fl oz) of boiling water with the lemon juice and sip. Add stevia if you like it sweet.

When? On rising, before breakfast.

Why? Drinking a large glass of warm water with fresh lemon assists hydration levels after a night's fast and boosts kidney function.

Note Drink this before brushing your teeth, to protect your gum health.

CHOOSE UP TO THREE PER DAY

★ Filter coffee, with a maximum of 50ml (2fl oz) of skimmed milk

★ Small 'skinny' cappuccino, made with skimmed milk (limit to 1 per day)

★ Single espresso   ★ English Breakfast tea   ★ Green tea

★ Louise's Thermogenic Tea – to make 1 litre (1¾ pints), steep 1 cinnamon stick, 1 mint teabag and 1 green-teabag in 1 litre (1¾ pints) of boiling water overnight. Serve ice-cold. Please remember that this tea contains caffeine, so do not drink it after 3pm, to ensure a good night's sleep.

UNLIMITED DRINKS PER DAY

★ Still mineral, spring or filter water

★ Herbal teas   ★ Fruit infusions

★ Still water flavoured with fresh cucumber, lemon, lime or orange slices, or mint

★ Chilled herbal teas

How much water you need depends on the amount of exercise you have done during the day, and you may wish to drink an additional 1 litre (1¾ pints) of water per day if you exercise heavily. The general target is a minimum of 2 litres (3½ pints) a day.

FORBIDDEN DRINKS

★ Any alcoholic drink, including 'slimline' drinks

★ Soda or diet soda, such as Diet Coke

★ Fruit juice (freshly squeezed or shop-bought)

★ Lattes   ★ Vegetable juices   ★ Coconut water

★ Any cordials – including sugar-free and 'No added sugar' options

★ Low-calorie hot-chocolate drinks

THE FOOD-PLAN RECIPES

★ All recipes serve one unless otherwise stated.

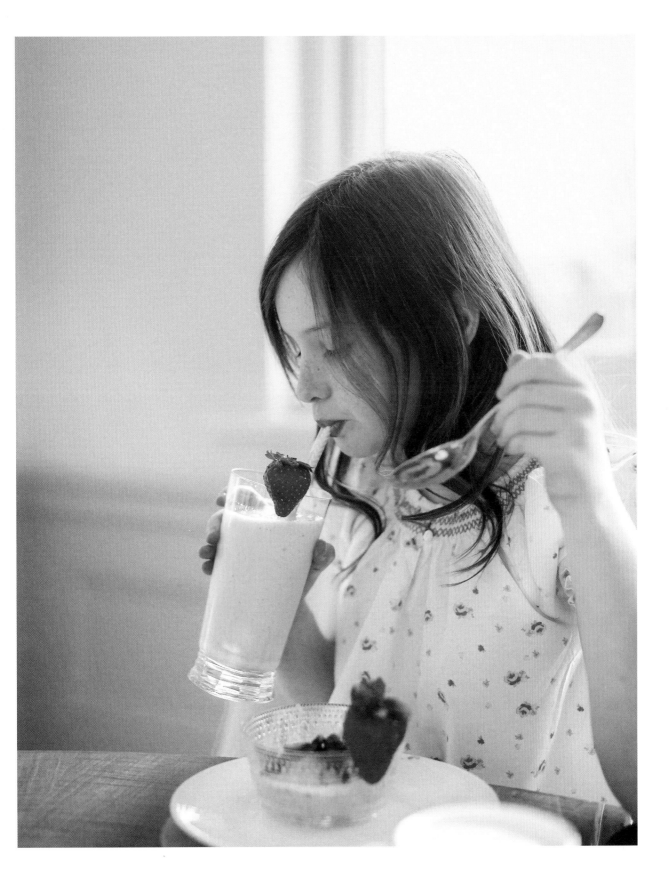

BREAKFASTS

Blueberry Pancakes & Hot Raspberry Sauce

1 tablespoon oat bran

1 tablespoon wholemeal flour

1 tablespoon dried skimmed milk

2 tablespoons soya milk

1 organic egg

¼ teaspoon vanilla paste

¼ teaspoon stevia

¼ teaspoon baking powder

¼ cup blueberries

1 teaspoon butter

Hot Raspberry Sauce:

½ cup raspberries, fresh or frozen

pinch of stevia

Combine the oat bran, flour and dried milk in a food processor or blender, then add the soya milk, egg, vanilla paste, stevia and baking powder. Blend for 30 seconds and then add the blueberries.

Melt the butter in a frying pan and pan-fry tablespoons of the batter to make the pancakes, turning them over when the mixture forms bubbles on the surface.

To make the hot raspberry sauce, cook the raspberries and stevia together gently in a saucepan for 2 minutes. Pour the sauce over the blueberry pancakes and enjoy.

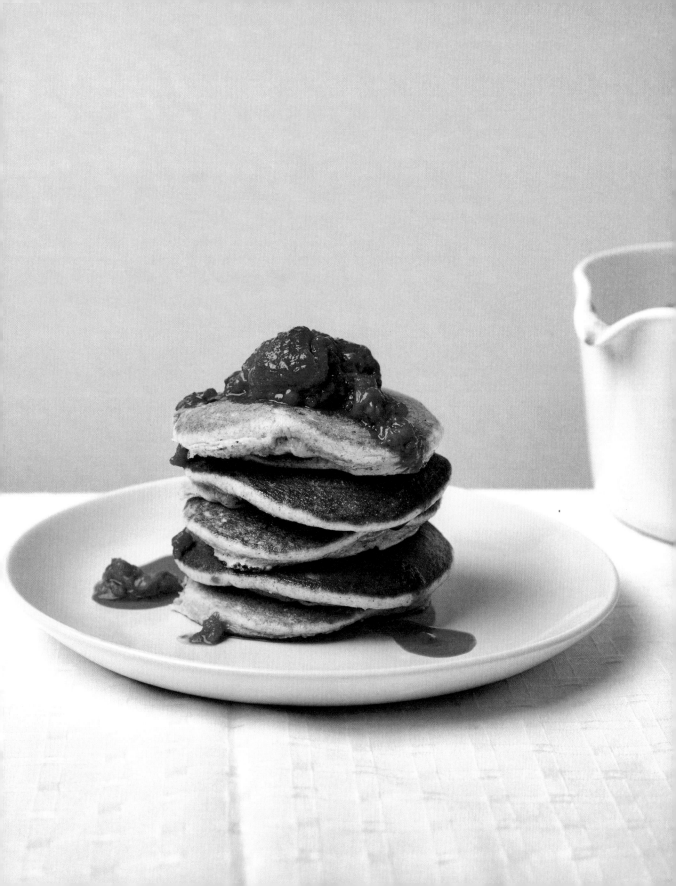

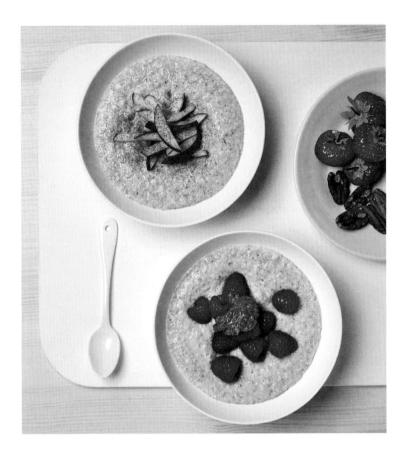

Vanilla Oat Bran Porridge

2 tablespoons oat bran

1½ cups semi-skimmed milk

1 teaspoon vanilla paste

pinch of salt

Toppings:

1 teaspoon cashew nut butter and a
handful of strawberries

1 teaspoon almond butter and a
handful of raspberries

ground cinnamon and apple slices

1 teaspoon cherry concentrate and
salted pecan nuts

Combine the oat bran with the milk, vanilla paste
and salt in a saucepan and simmer for 2 minutes
until the mixture bubbles and turns creamy.

Serve with your chosen topping.

*My oat bran porridge is lower-carb than normal
or 'healthy halo' porridge. You need less oat bran
than standard oats to make a deliciously creamy
high-fibre version. For a lower-carb version, use
either lactose-free milk or soya milk, and add a
pinch of stevia for more sweetness.*

*We can now afford to adorn the porridge with
beautiful, flavoursome toppings. Think flavour –
and make it a feast for the eyes too!*

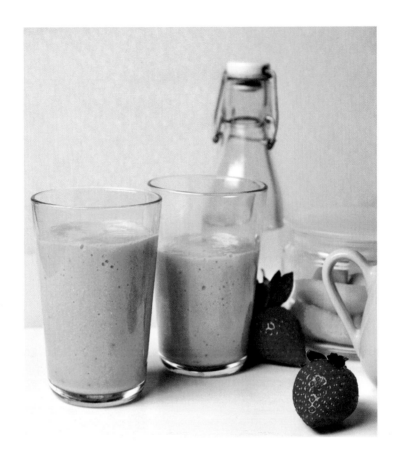

Mango & Strawberry Smoothie

⅓ cup fresh or frozen mango cubes

1 cup strawberries, chopped

1 tablespoon oat bran

150g (5½oz) low-fat Greek yogurt

1 cup water

Blend the mango, strawberries, oat bran, yogurt and water together, ideally using a powerful blender, for 1 minute, or until smooth.

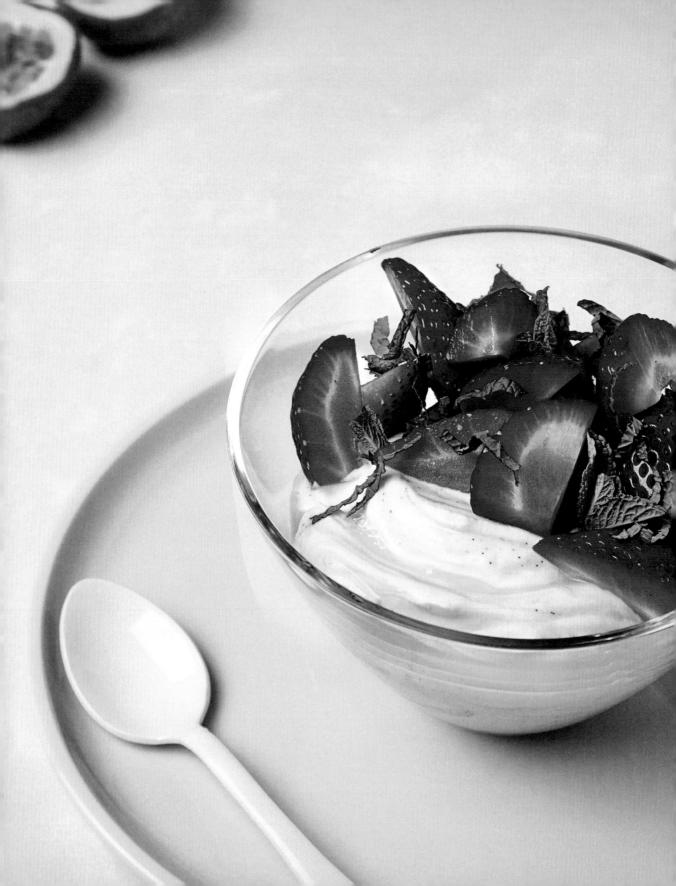

Strawberry Mint Salad with Passion Fruit Yogurt

2 cups ripe strawberries, sliced

handful of mint leaves, finely sliced

juice of ½ lime

150g (5½oz) low-fat Greek yogurt

juice of 2 passion fruit

½ teaspoon vanilla paste

¼ teaspoon stevia (optional)

Combine the strawberries with the mint in a bowl and drizzle with the lime juice.

Serve with the Greek yogurt mixed with the passion fruit juice, vanilla paste and stevia, if using.

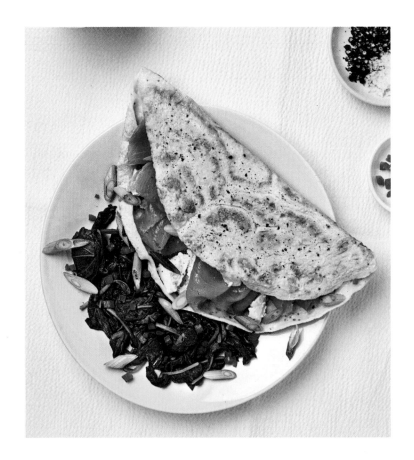

Beloved Omelette

2 organic eggs

25g (1oz) goats' cheese

25g (1oz) smoked salmon

2 cups spinach

1 teaspoon butter

spring onions, sliced, to garnish

chopped fresh red chilli,
to taste (optional)

sea salt and ground black pepper

Whisk the eggs well and pour into a nonstick omelette pan set over a high heat. Cook for 1 minute then sprinkle over the goats' cheese and lay the smoked salmon on top. Fold the omelette in half and season to taste.

Sauté the spinach in the butter. Garnish with the sliced spring onion, and chilli, if liked, then serve beside the omelette.

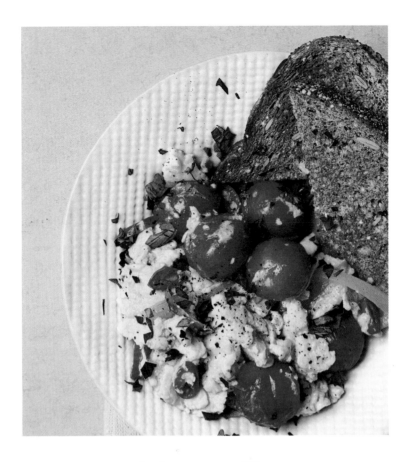

Messy Eggs

1 teaspoon butter

6 cherry tomatoes

½ red chilli, deseeded and sliced

½ yellow or red pepper, cored, deseeded and sliced

2 large organic eggs

chopped flat leaf parsley or coriander leaves, to garnish (optional)

1 thin slice of wholegrain or soda bread, toasted

sea salt and ground black pepper

Melt the butter in a pan over a medium heat and pan-fry the tomatoes, chilli and pepper in the butter.

Add the eggs, reduce the heat and scramble together slowly. Season to taste and garnish with the parsley or coriander, if using, and serve with the toast.

Butter Peaches with Vanilla Ricotta Cream

1 peach, stoned and quartered

½ teaspoon butter, softened

100g (3½oz) low-fat Greek yogurt

50g (1¾oz) low-fat ricotta cheese

½ teaspoon vanilla paste

4 pecan nuts, roasted and roughly chopped

Brush the peach quarters with butter and cook under a medium grill or in a frying pan until golden and fragrant.

Stir the yogurt, ricotta and vanilla paste together in a bowl until well combined and serve topped with the warm peaches and sprinkled with the pecans.

Apple, Cinnamon & Walnut Bircher

1 apple, peel on, grated

150g (5½oz) low-fat Greek yogurt

1 level teaspoon ground cinnamon

2 tablespoons oat bran

6 walnuts

Mix the apple with the yogurt, cinnamon and oat bran. Leave to soak overnight in the fridge.

Toast the walnuts in a dry frying pan for a minute or two. Serve the Bircher with the warm, toasted walnuts on top.

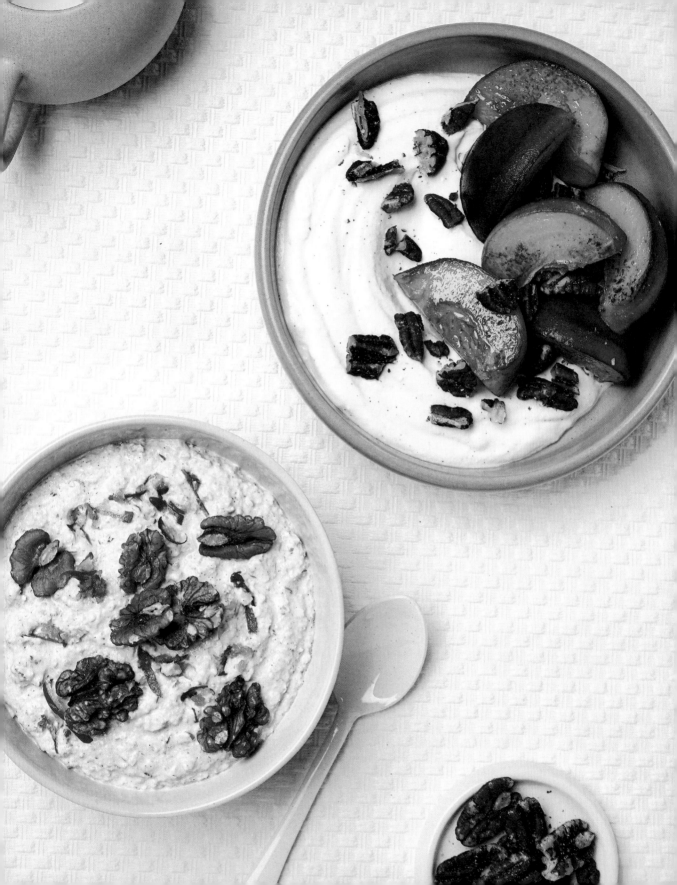

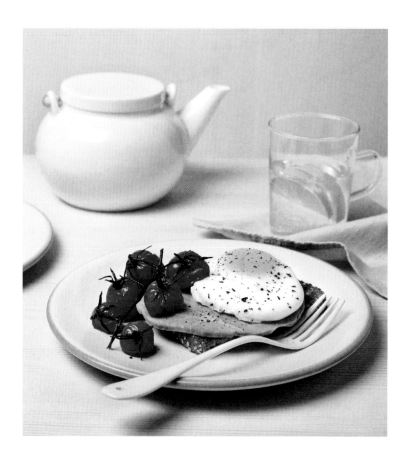

Skinny Benedict

6 cherry tomatoes on the vine

1 teaspoon olive oil

1 thick slice of premium ham

1 slice of wholegrain bread, toasted

1 organic egg, poached or soft-boiled

sea salt and ground black pepper

Pan-fry the tomatoes in the olive oil over a low–medium heat for 6 minutes, or until soft.

Place the ham on the toast. Top with the poached or soft-boiled egg, season to taste and serve with the tomatoes alongside.

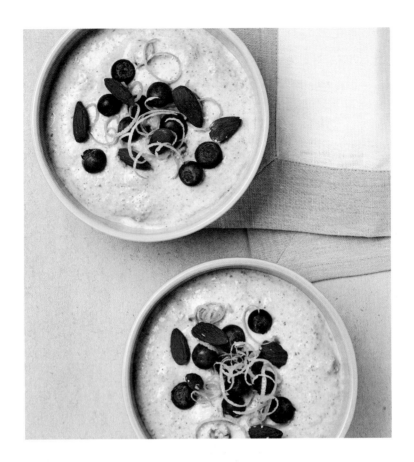

Lemon Blueberry Bircher with Toasted Almonds

150g (5½oz) low-fat Greek yogurt

2 tablespoons oat bran

4 tablespoons skimmed milk

¼ teaspoon stevia

½ teaspoon vanilla paste

6 whole almonds

½ cup blueberries

½ teaspoon pared lemon zest

Mix the yogurt together in a bowl with the oat bran, milk, stevia and vanilla paste. Leave to soak in the fridge overnight.

Toast the almonds in a dry frying pan for a minute or two.

Serve the Bircher, with the toasted almonds, blueberries and pared lemon zest on top.

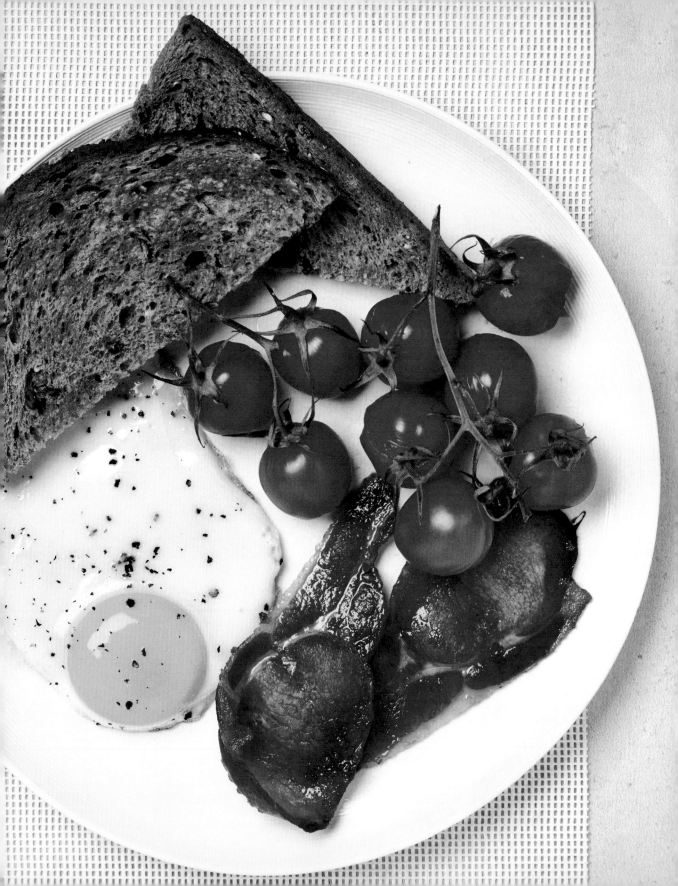

Fit Fry-up

2 thick, lean bacon rashers

½ teaspoon butter

1 large organic egg

10 cherry tomatoes on the vine

½ teaspoon olive oil

sea salt and ground black pepper

1 slice of wholemeal bread, toasted

Cook the bacon under the grill. Melt the butter in a frying pan and fry the egg. Now pan-fry the tomatoes in the olive oil over a medium heat for 2 minutes, or until soft. Season to taste and serve with the toast.

Eggs & Soldiers with Prosciutto-wrapped Asparagus

2 large organic eggs

2 slices of lean prosciutto

6 asparagus spears, lightly steamed

1 thin slice of wholegrain bread, toasted

sea salt and ground black pepper

Soft-boil the eggs.

Meanwhile, wrap the prosciutto around the asparagus spears.

Cut the toast into soldiers. Serve the eggs with the soldiers and prosciutto-wrapped asparagus.

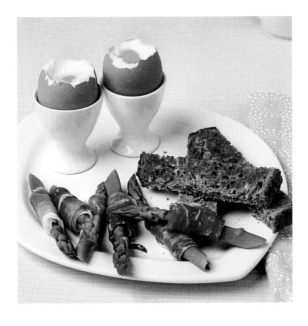

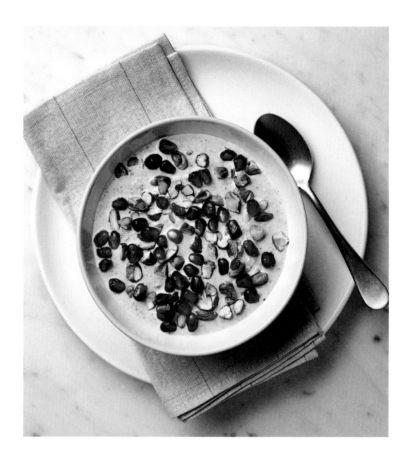

Bejewelled Pomegranate & Pistachio Bircher

150g (5½oz) low-fat Greek yogurt

2 tablespoons oat bran

4 tablespoons skimmed milk

¼ teaspoon stevia, or to taste

1 teaspoon vanilla paste

1 tablespoon pistachio nuts, chopped

2 tablespoons pomegranate seeds

Mix together the yogurt, oat bran, milk, stevia and vanilla paste in a bowl and leave to soak overnight in the fridge.

Serve topped with the pistachios and pomegranate seeds.

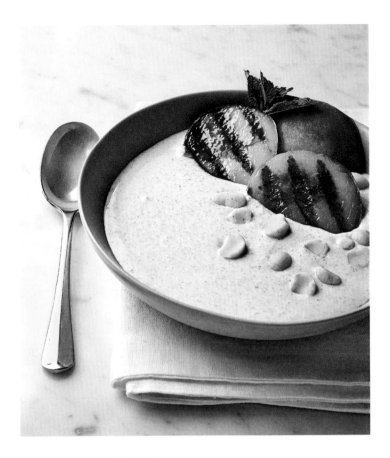

Grilled Nectarine with Vanilla Bircher

150g (5½oz) low-fat Greek yogurt

¼ teaspoon stevia

1 teaspoon vanilla paste

4 tablespoons skimmed milk

2 tablespoons oat bran

1 ripe nectarine, stoned

5 macadamia nuts, toasted

mint sprig, to garnish

Mix together the yogurt, stevia, vanilla paste, milk and oat bran in a bowl. Leave to soak overnight in the fridge.

Slice the nectarine in half or into slices and grill or griddle it until caramelized.

Serve the vanilla bircher topped with the warm nectarine and toasted macadamia nuts and garnished with a mint sprig.

Milly's Strawberry &
Oat Bran Bircher

150g (5½oz) low-fat Greek yogurt

¾ cup ripe strawberries, sliced

2 tablespoons oat bran

pinch of stevia, or to taste

1 teaspoon vanilla paste

dash of skimmed milk

1 fig, cut into sixths

1 tablespoon hazelnuts, toasted

Mix together the yogurt, sliced strawberries, oat bran, stevia and vanilla paste and leave to soak overnight in the fridge.

To serve, loosen the bircher with the milk and top with the fig pieces and warm hazelnuts for crunch.

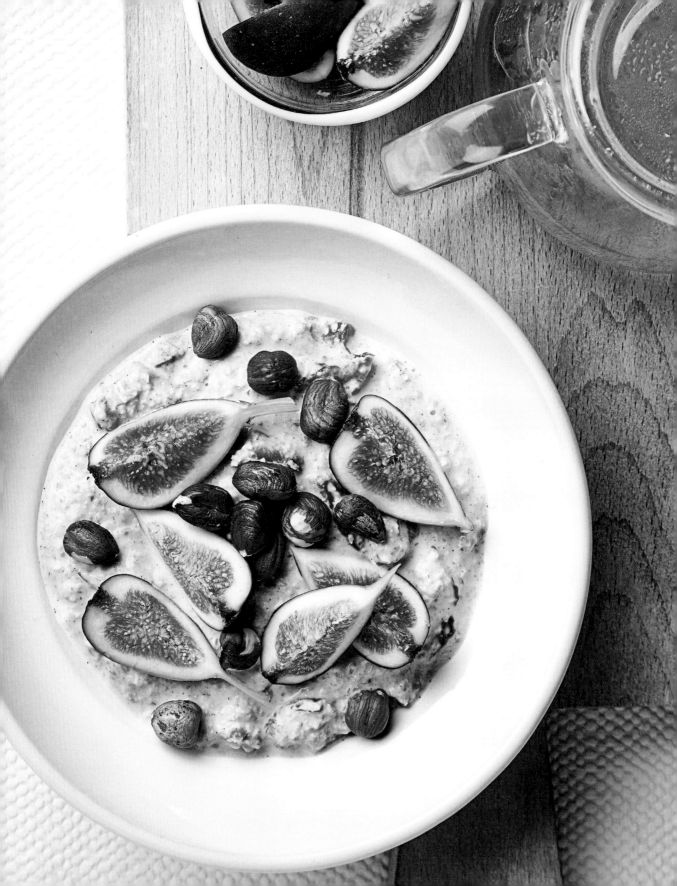

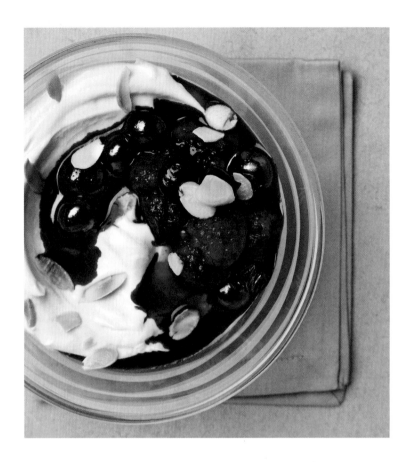

Yogurt & Summer Berry Compote with Almonds

½ cup fresh blueberries and ½ cup fresh raspberries (or 1 cup frozen summer berries)

½ teaspoon stevia

150g (5½oz) low-fat Greek yogurt

few flaked almonds, toasted

Place the berries in a saucepan, add the stevia and simmer over a low heat for 4 minutes. Leave to cool for 10 minutes (or make ahead and chill).

Serve the compote with the Greek yogurt, topped with the toasted almonds.

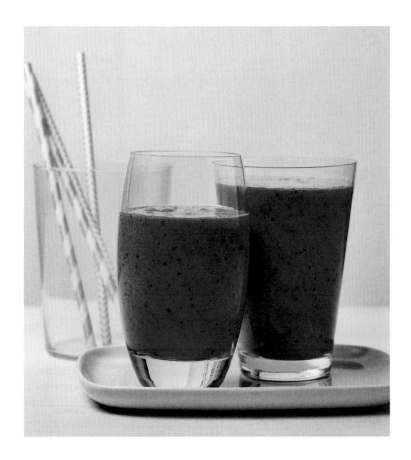

Vitality Smoothie

150g (5½oz) low-fat Greek yogurt

1 cup frozen summer berries

½ cup fresh blueberries

1 tablespoon oat bran

½ teaspoon stevia

up to 300ml (10fl oz) water

Blend the yogurt with the frozen berries and blueberries, the oat bran, stevia and some of the water, ideally using a powerful blender, for 1 minute, or until smooth. Add as much of the remaining water to reach your desired consistency.

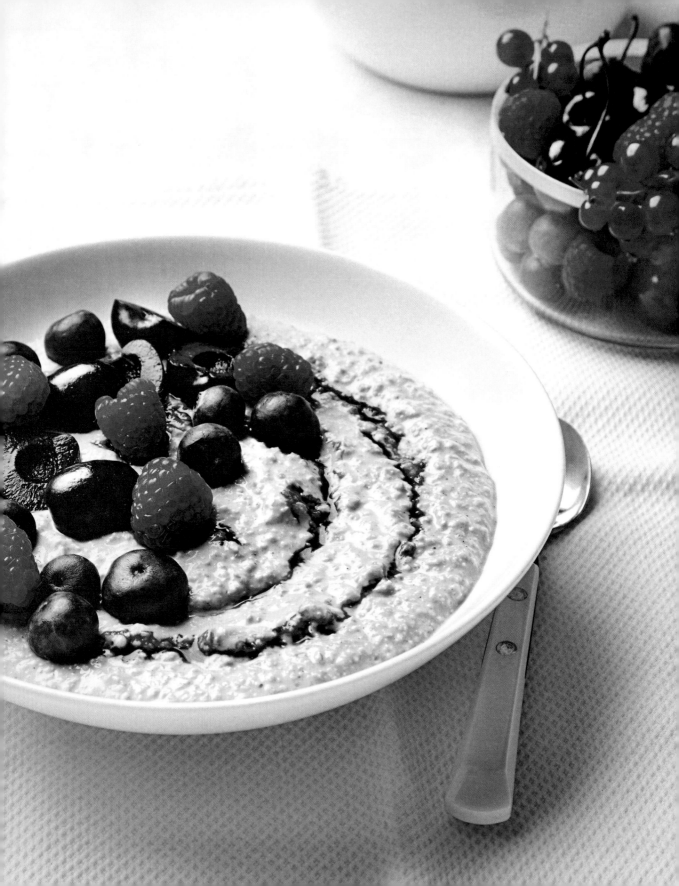

Super Cherry Bircher

150g (5½oz) low-fat Greek yogurt

2 tablespoons oat bran

½ teaspoon vanilla paste

½ cup skimmed milk

30ml (1fl oz) concentrated cherry juice

½ teaspoon stevia

1 teaspoon cherry concentrate

1 cup fresh cherries, raspberries or blueberries

Mix together the yogurt, oat bran, vanilla paste, milk, cherry juice and stevia. Leave to soak overnight.

Serve the bircher with the cherry concentrate drizzled on top and cherries, raspberries or blueberries scattered over.

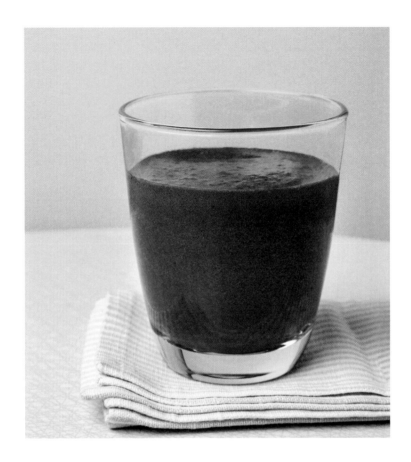

Good Morning Smoothie

1 scoop sugar-free chocolate
protein powder

1 shot of cooled espresso
(you can also freeze espresso shots
in advance)

½ teaspoon pure cocoa powder

½ banana (you can peel, halve and
freeze these in advance too)

up to 300ml (10fl oz) semi-skimmed milk

Blend the protein powder with the
espresso, cocoa powder, banana and
some of the milk, ideally using a powerful
blender, for 30 seconds, or until smooth.
Add as much of the remaining milk to
reach your desired consistency.

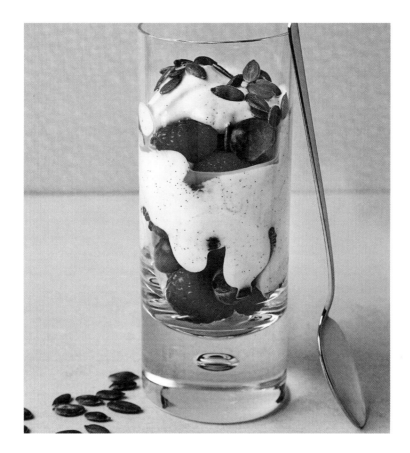

Anydae Sundae

150g (5½oz) low-fat Greek yogurt

75ml (2½fl oz) skimmed milk

½ teaspoon vanilla paste

¼ teaspoon stevia, or to taste
(optional)

handful of blueberries

handful of raspberries

juice of 2 passion fruit

1 teaspoon sunflower or pumpkin
seeds, toasted if you wish

Loosen the yogurt with the milk and add the vanilla paste. Add the stevia to taste, if using.

Layer the yogurt in a serving glass with the blueberries and raspberries.

Serve with the passion fruit juice squeezed over and sprinkled with the sunflower or pumpkin seeds.

SNACKS

Cinnamon Orange with Vanilla Yogurt

100g (3½oz) low-fat Greek yogurt

½ teaspoon stevia

1 teaspoon vanilla paste

1 orange (or ½ regular orange and ½ blood orange)

sprinkle of ground cinnamon

Mix together the yogurt in a bowl with the stevia and vanilla paste.

Peel and slice the orange, removing as much of the pith as possible.

Sprinkle the sweetened, flavoured yogurt with the cinnamon and serve with the orange slices.

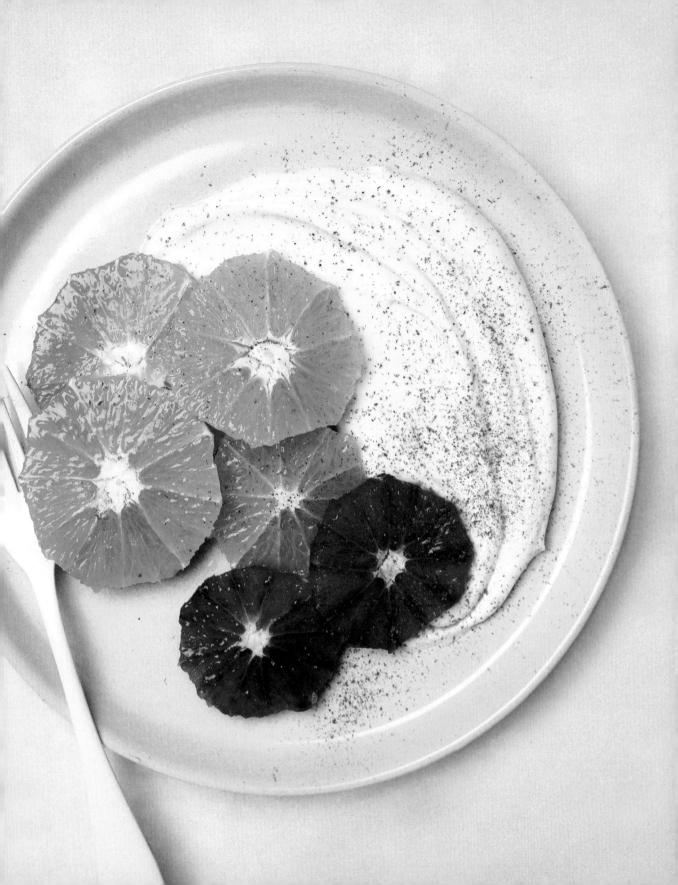

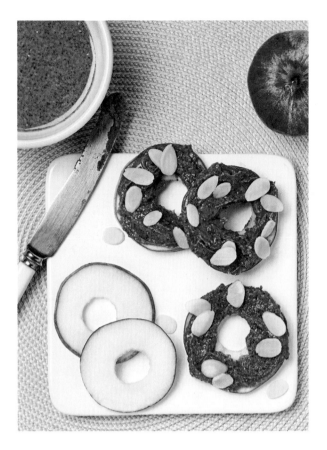

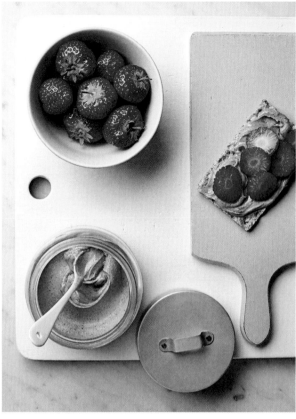

Apple & Almond Butter Doughnuts

1 apple, cored and sliced widthways

1 heaped tablespoon sugar-free almond butter

1 teaspoon flaked almonds, toasted

Spread 3 slices of apple with the almond butter then sprinkle with the toasted almonds.

Cashew & Strawberry Crunch

1 crispbread, such as Ryvita

1 tablespoon sugar-free cashew nut butter

handful of strawberries, sliced

Spread the crispbread with the cashew nut butter and serve sprinkled with the strawberries.

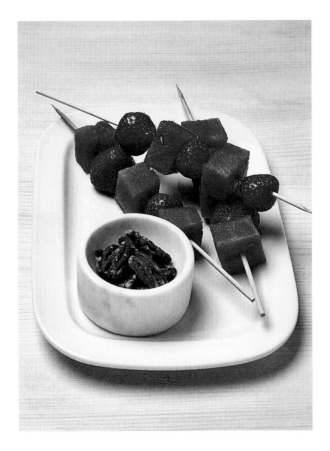

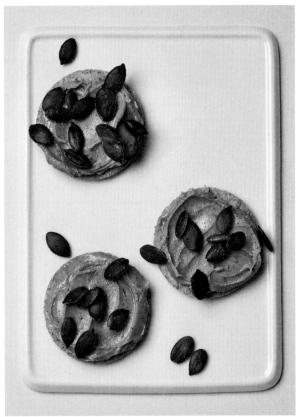

Watermelon & Strawberry Skewers with Pecans

1 cup strawberries

1 cup cubed watermelon

8 pecan nuts, toasted

Slide the strawberries and watermelon cubes onto kebab skewers and serve with the toasted pecans.

Peanut Butter & Pumpkin Seed Oatcakes

3 mini oatcakes

1 tablespoon sugar-free peanut butter (ideally Whole Earth)

few pumpkin seeds

Spread the oatcakes with the peanut butter, then sprinkle with the pumpkin seeds.

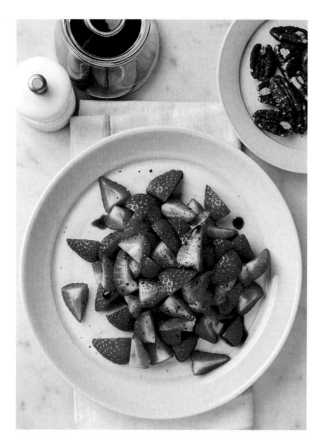

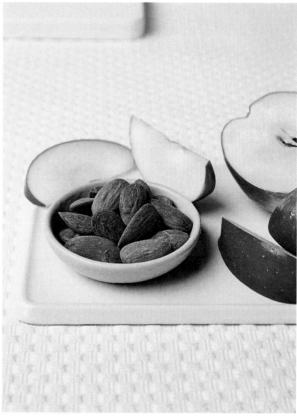

Balsamic Strawberries & Salted Pecans

12 strawberries

1 tablespoon really good balsamic vinegar

pinch of ground black pepper

6 salted, roasted pecan nuts

Cut the strawberries into quarters and drizzle with the balsamic vinegar, then season with the black pepper. Serve with the pecan nuts on the side.

Apple & Almonds

1 crunchy apple

20 almonds

Tajín seasoning powder (optional)

Apple with almonds is such a simple, grab-and-go snack. If you're at home, core and thinly slice the apple and sprinkle it with toasted, flaked almonds.

If you love chilli and lime, try seasoning the apple with Tajín powder, available from Mexican stores online. *Amazing!*

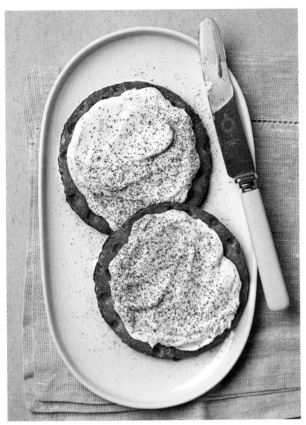

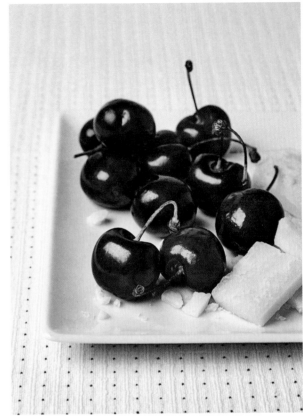

Ricotta Cinnamon Crunch

75g (2¾oz) low-fat ricotta cheese

pinch of stevia

½ teaspoon ground cinnamon

2 rye crispbreads or oatcakes

Mix the ricotta together with the stevia
and cinnamon in a small bowl. Spread over
the rye crispbreads or oatcakes.

Cherries & Parmesan

10 cherries

25g (1oz) good Parmesan cheese, cut into chunks

Combine sweet cherries with little chunks of
Parmesan for a simple and quick taste sensation.

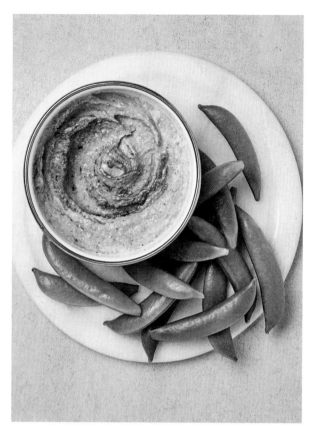

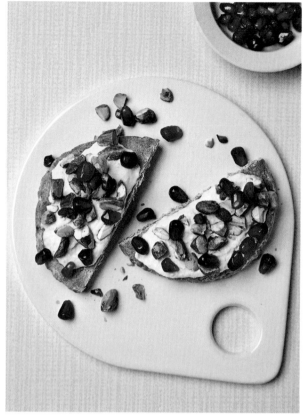

Hummus & Sugarsnaps

1 teaspoon smoked chilli paste

2 tablespoons hummus

30 sugarsnap peas

Combine the chilli paste and hummus and enjoy as a dip for the raw, sweet sugarsnaps.

Hummus & Pomegranate Pitta

1 wholemeal mini pitta

1 heaped tablespoon hummus

1 tablespoon chopped pistachios

1 tablespoon pomegranate seeds

Warm the pitta in the toaster, spread with the hummus and sprinkle with the pistachios and pomegranate seeds.

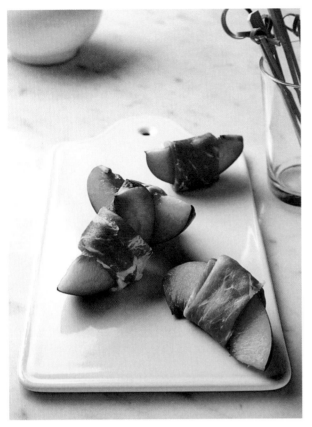

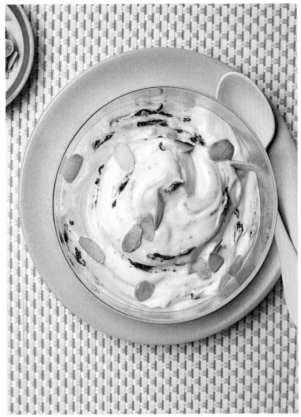

Nectarine Prosciutto Skewers

1 ripe nectarine

4 slices of lean prosciutto

Cut the nectarine into quarters and wrap
each quarter with a slice of prosciutto.

Almond Yogurt

2 teaspoons sugar-free almond butter

100g (3½oz) low-fat Greek yogurt

½ teaspoon stevia

1 tablespoon flaked almonds, toasted

Mix the almond butter into the yogurt along
with the stevia. Serve sprinkled with the
toasted almonds.

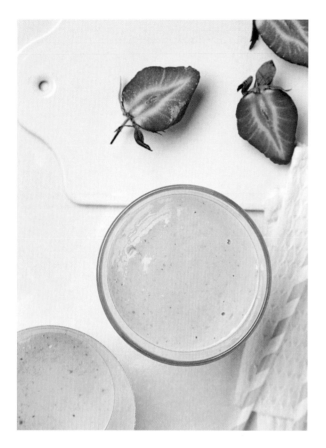

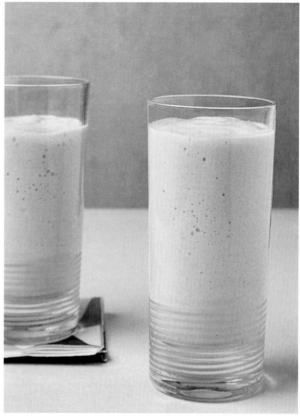

Strawberry Vanilla Smoothie

100g (3½oz) strawberries

100g (3½oz) low-fat Greek yogurt

1 teaspoon vanilla paste

1 heaped tablespoon oat bran

100–200ml (3½–7fl oz) skimmed milk

Blend all the ingredients together, ideally
using a powerful blender, for 1 minute,
or until smooth. Adjust the amount of milk
to your preferred consistency.

Vanilla, Peach & Almond Smoothie

8 segments of fresh or frozen peach

100g (3½oz) low-fat Greek yogurt

½ teaspoon vanilla or almond extract

½ teaspoon stevia

½ tablespoon ground almonds

100ml (3½fl oz) skimmed milk

Blend all the ingredients together, ideally
using a powerful blender, for 1 minute, or until
smooth. Adjust the amount of milk to your
preferred consistency.

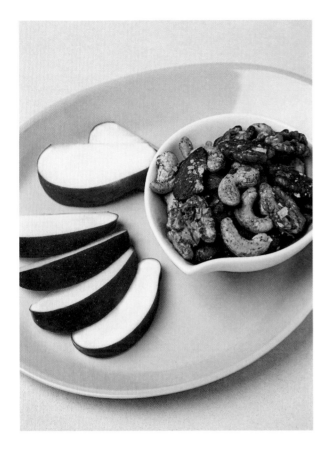

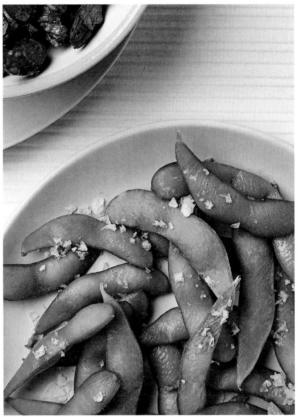

Cinnamon Nuts

Makes 8 servings; a serving is ¼ cup plus an apple

1 organic egg white

½ cup each almonds, cashews, pecan nuts and walnuts

¾ teaspoon stevia | ½ teaspoon sea salt

2 teaspoons ground cinnamon | 1 apple per serving

Preheat the oven to 150°C (300°F), Gas Mark 2. Whip the egg white, then fold in the nuts, the stevia, half the sea salt and half the cinnamon. Throw onto a lightly oiled baking sheet and bake for 15 minutes, stirring every 5 minutes. Remove from the oven and stir in the rest of the sea salt and cinnamon.

Edamame Beans & Sea Salt

25 frozen edamame beans

sea salt

Defrost the edamame beans in hot water for 5 minutes. Drain thoroughly and then season with the salt.

A great, simple, portable snack.

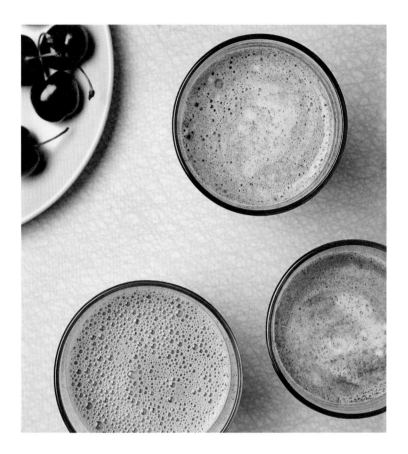

Black Cherry Smoothie

100g (3½oz) low-fat Greek yogurt

1 cup cherries, fresh or frozen

100–200ml (3½–7fl oz) skimmed milk

1 tablespoon cherry concentrate

Blend all the ingredients together, ideally using a powerful blender, for 1 minute, or until smooth. Adjust the amount of milk to your desired consistency.

Vanilla Cinnamon Smoothie

100g (3½oz) low-fat Greek yogurt

1 teaspoon vanilla paste

½ teaspoon ground cinnamon

100–200ml (3½–7fl oz) skimmed milk

Blend all the ingredients together, ideally using a powerful blender, for 30 seconds, or until smooth. Adjust the amount of milk to your desired consistency.

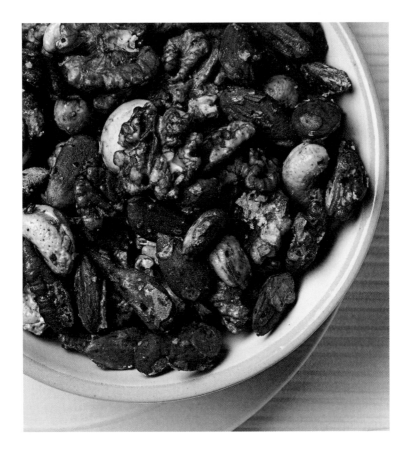

Chipotle & Rosemary Salted Nuts

Makes 8 servings; a serving is ¼ cup plus 12 cherries

1 organic egg white

½ cup almonds

½ cup cashews

½ cup pecan nuts

½ cup walnuts

1 teaspoon stevia

½ teaspoon sea salt

½ teaspoon chipotle powder

1 teaspoon chopped fresh rosemary

12 cherries per serving

Preheat the oven to 150°C (300°F), Gas Mark 2.

Whip the egg white, then fold in the nuts, the stevia, half the salt, the chipotle powder and half the rosemary.

Throw onto a lightly oiled baking sheet and bake for 15 minutes, stirring every 5 minutes.

Remove from the oven and stir in the rest of the salt and rosemary.

LUNCHES

Tofu Samui Soup

1 stick of lemongrass

a little fresh ginger, peeled and finely chopped

250ml (9fl oz) good vegetable stock

1 cup mangetout, sliced diagonally

½ red pepper, sliced

1 cup oyster mushrooms

4 stems of tenderstem broccoli

2 tablespoons shelled edamame beans

200g (7oz) firm smoked tofu, chopped

1 red chilli, deseeded and sliced

1 tablespoon reduced-salt soy sauce

chopped coriander leaves or Thai basil, to garnish

Bash the lemongrass to release the flavour then place it in a saucepan with the ginger and stock. Simmer over a medium heat for 5 minutes and then remove the lemongrass and ginger with a slotted spoon.

Add the mangetout, red pepper, mushrooms, broccoli, edamame beans, tofu, chilli and soy sauce to the stock and simmer for 4 minutes, or until the vegetables are al dente. Garnish with the coriander or basil.

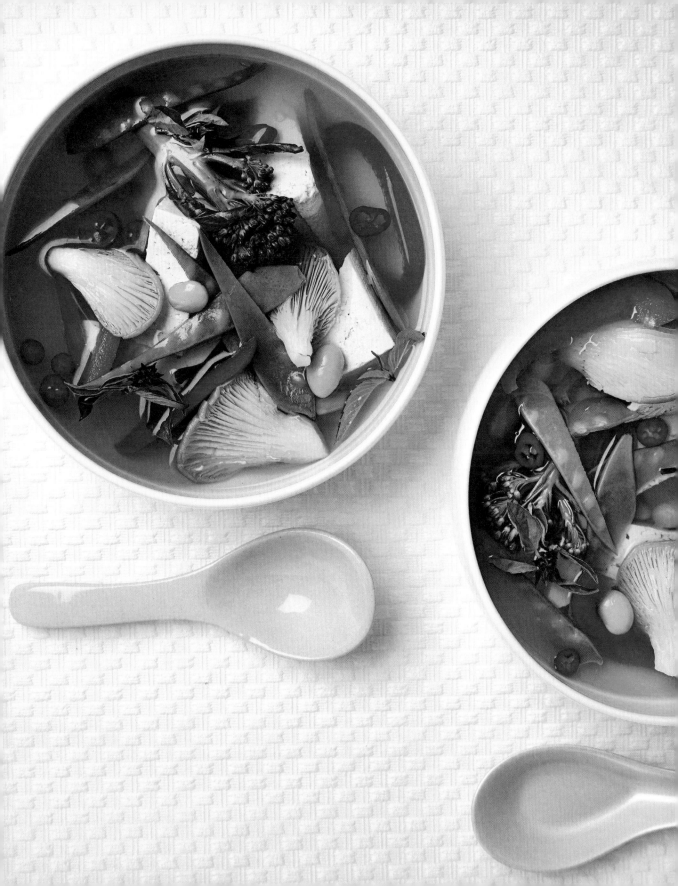

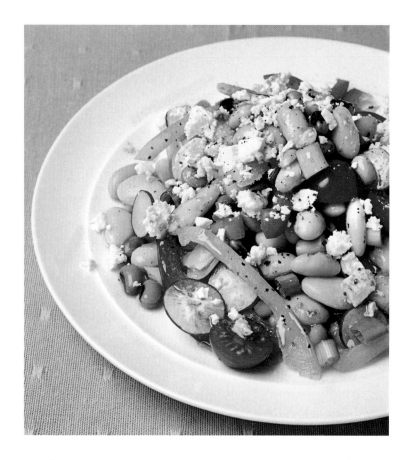

Three Bean & Feta Salad

¼ cup canned cannellini beans

¼ cup canned butter beans

¼ cup canned black-eye beans

4 spring onions, chopped

½ yellow pepper, cored, deseeded and sliced

½ red pepper, cored, deseeded and sliced

4 radishes, sliced

6 cherry tomatoes, halved

1 teaspoon olive oil

1 teaspoon green pesto

50g (1¾oz) feta cheese, crumbled

Mix together all the beans in a bowl. Add the spring onions, peppers, radishes, tomatoes, olive oil and pesto and toss to combine.

Sprinkle with the feta and serve.

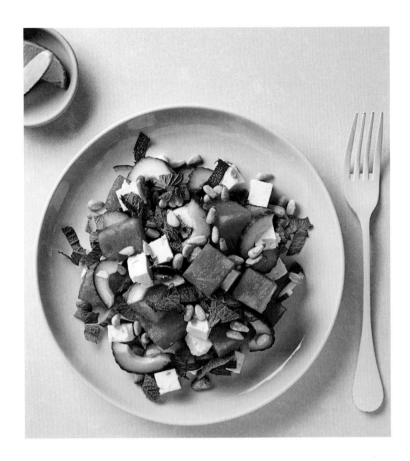

Summer Feta Salad

¼ small watermelon

75g (2¾oz) feta cheese, cubed

¼ cucumber, deseeded and sliced

handful of mint, chopped

juice of ½ lime

1 tablespoon pine nuts, toasted

Cut the watermelon into chunks, then add the cubed feta, cucumber and mint. Dress with the lime juice and sprinkle with the pine nuts.

Goats' Cheese & Beetroot Salad

75g (2¾oz) soft goats' cheese

2 handfuls of young leaf spinach

7.5cm (3 inches) cucumber, sliced

12 cherry tomatoes, halved

1 small ready-cooked beetroot, sliced

1 cup broccoli florets, blanched

1 teaspoon pine nuts, toasted

1 teaspoon walnut oil

juice of ½ lemon

sea salt and ground black pepper

Add the goats' cheese to the salad of spinach, cucumber, tomatoes, beetroot and broccoli. Top with the warm, toasted pine nuts. Dress with the walnut oil, lemon juice and salt and pepper.

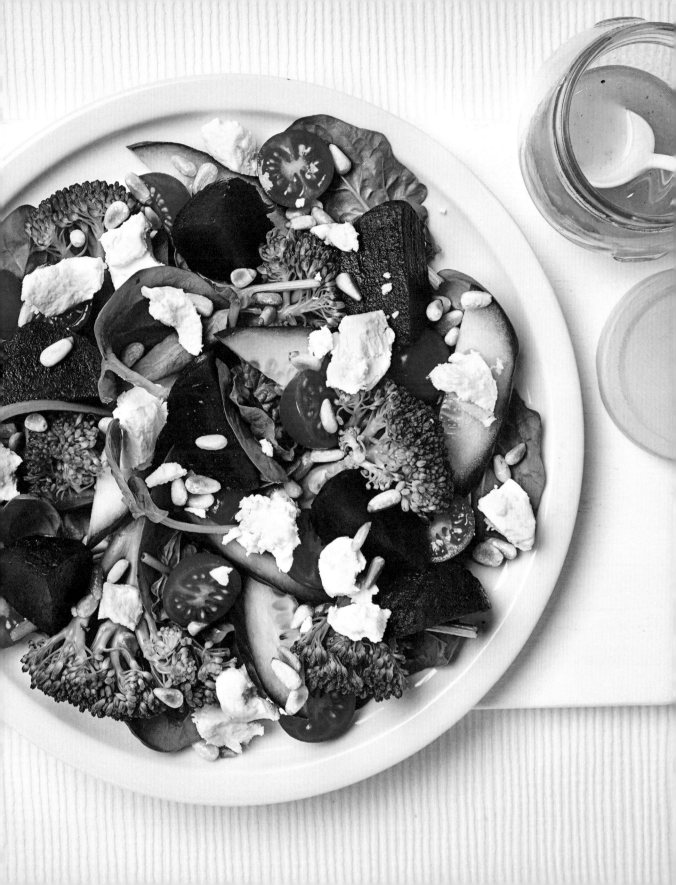

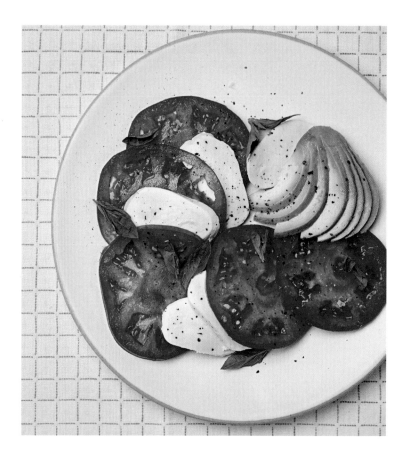

Classic Tricolour Salad

1 large beef tomato

1 ball of reduced-fat buffalo
mozzarella cheese

¼ ripe avocado

few basil leaves

1 tablespoon good balsamic vinegar

sea salt and ground black pepper

Slice the tomato, mozzarella and
avocado and arrange on a plate
with the basil.

Drizzle with the balsamic vinegar
and season with salt and pepper.

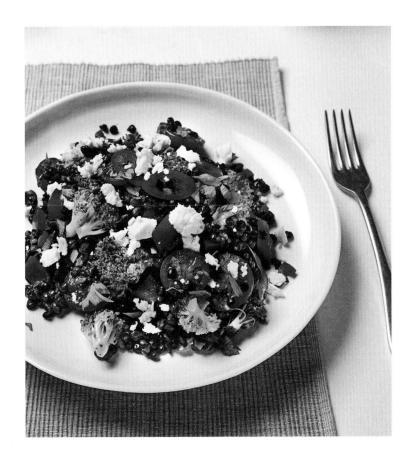

Louise's Lovely Lentils

¾ cup ready-cooked Beluga lentils, cold or warmed according to your preference

12 cherry tomatoes, halved

½ red pepper, cored, deseeded and chopped

½ red chilli, deseeded and chopped

1 cup broccoli florets, blanched

handful of flat leaf parsley, chopped

1 tablespoon good balsamic vinegar

1 tablespoon olive oil

50g (1¾oz) goats' cheese, crumbled

sea salt and ground black pepper

Mix together the lentils, tomatoes, pepper, chilli, broccoli and parsley in a bowl. Drizzle over the balsamic vinegar and olive oil and season to taste. Top with the crumbled goats' cheese to serve.

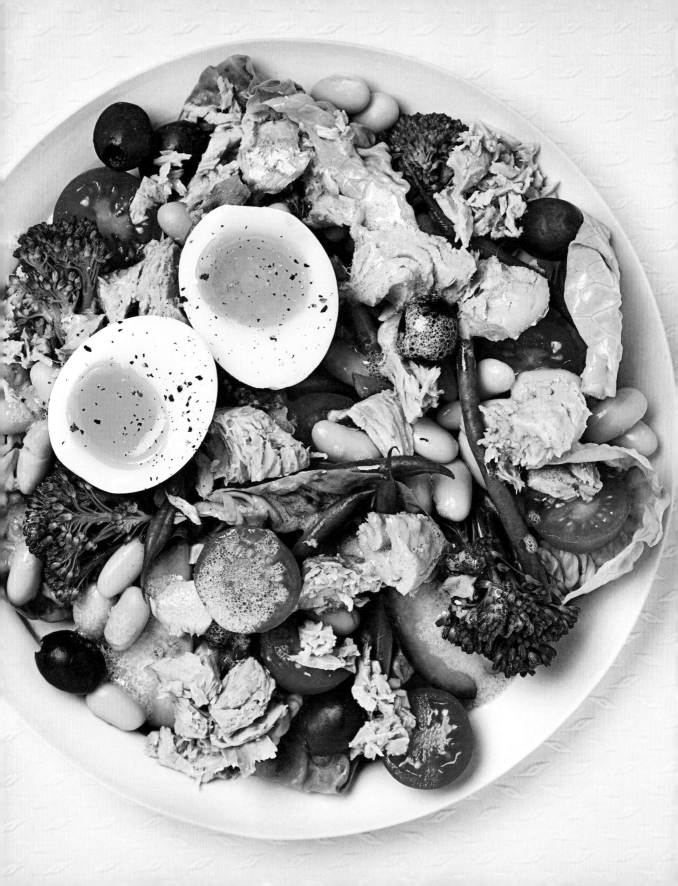

Slinky Niçoise

1 baby gem lettuce

1 cup French beans, blanched

75g (2¾oz) canned tuna

6 black olives, pitted

6 cherry tomatoes, halved

5cm (2 inches) cucumber, sliced

1 cup broccoli florets, blanched

¼ cup canned cannellini beans

1 tablespoon olive oil

1 teaspoon Dijon mustard

juice of ½ lemon

ground black pepper

1 soft-boiled organic egg, halved

Combine the lettuce, French beans, tuna, olives, tomatoes, cucumber, broccoli and cannellini beans.

Dress with the olive oil, mustard, lemon juice and black pepper and top with the soft-boiled egg halves.

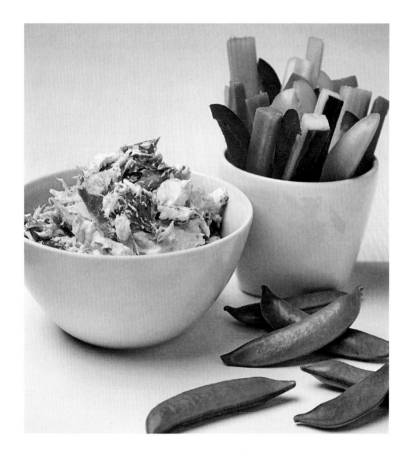

Smoked Mackerel Crudités

75g (2¾oz) smoked mackerel
fillets, flaked

juice of ½ lemon

50g (1¾oz) low-fat Greek yogurt

50g (1¾oz) low-fat cream cheese

handful of flat leaf parsley, chopped
(optional)

ground black pepper

crudités of cucumber sticks, sliced red
and yellow peppers, celery sticks and
sugarsnap peas

Blend the smoked mackerel, lemon juice, yogurt, cream cheese and black pepper with a fork. Stir in the parsley, if using.

Serve with the vegetable crudités.

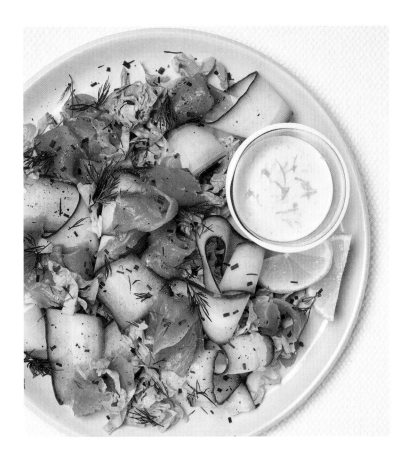

Oak-smoked Salmon, Dill & Cucumber Salad

1 cucumber (skin on)

1 little gem lettuce, finely chopped

75g (2¾oz) oak-smoked salmon

a little fresh dill and chives, chopped

1 tablespoon low-fat Greek yogurt

juice of ½ lemon

½ teaspoon grated lemon zest

sea salt and ground black pepper

lemon wedges, to garnish

Use a vegetable peeler to peel the cucumber into ribbons, leaving the inner seeds in, then combine with the lettuce and smoked salmon. Sprinkle over the herbs.

For the dressing, combine the yogurt with the lemon juice and zest, and then season to taste.

Serve the salad with the dressing on the side to drizzle over and lemon wedges to garnish.

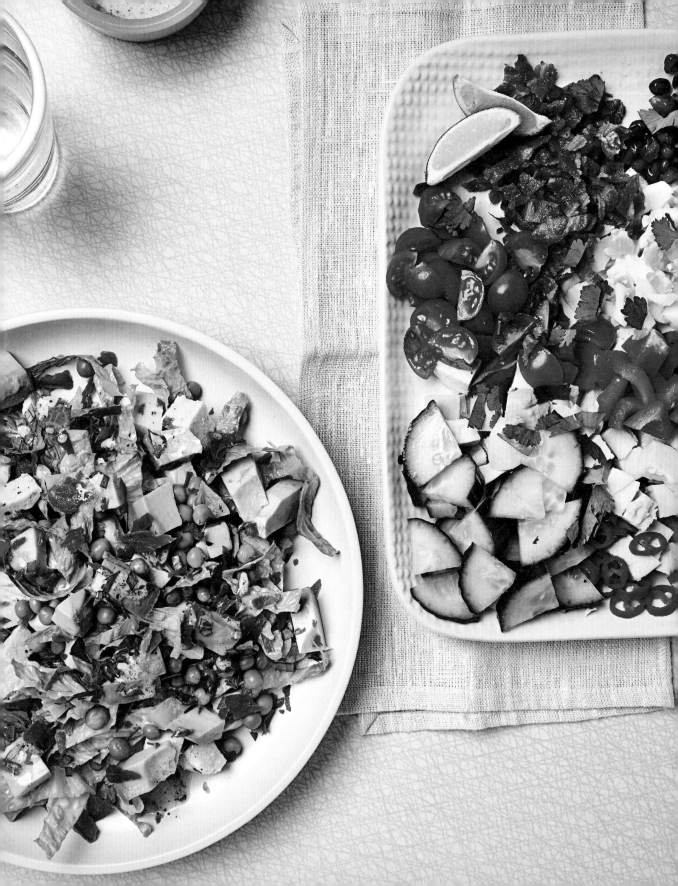

Pommy Cobb Salad

75g (2¾oz) cooked chicken breast

10cm (4 inches) cucumber, quartered lengthways and thickly sliced

8 cherry tomatoes, quartered

½ red pepper, cored, deseeded and chopped

½ red chilli, deseeded and sliced

handful of fresh coriander leaves, roughly chopped

seeds of ½ pomegranate

1 hard-boiled organic egg, chopped

2 rashers of cooked smoked streaky bacon, finely chopped

2 teaspoons mild olive oil

lime wedges, to garnish

Chop the chicken breast finely, then arrange on a plate with the cucumber, tomatoes, pepper, chilli, coriander leaves, pomegranate seeds, chopped egg and bacon.

Dress with the olive oil and serve garnished with lime wedges for squeezing over.

Best Bistro Salad

1 little gem lettuce

handful of fresh tarragon

handful of flat leaf parsley

½ avocado, cubed

2 slices of lean prosciutto, baked and chopped

1 cup frozen peas, cooked

100g (3½oz) cooked chicken breast, chopped

1 tablespoon olive oil

1 tablespoon lemon juice or white wine vinegar

1 teaspoon Dijon mustard

crushed garlic, to taste

sea salt and ground black pepper

Finely chop the lettuce, tarragon and parsley and place in a serving dish. Add the cubed avocado, chopped baked prosciutto, cooked peas and chopped cooked chicken.

Mix the olive oil, vinegar, mustard and crushed garlic together, season to taste and drizzle over the salad.

Chilli Chicken Salad

125g (4½oz) cooked chicken breast, shredded

5 handfuls of young leaf spinach

4 radishes, sliced

4 baby plum tomatoes, halved

10cm (4 inches) cucumber, halved lengthways and sliced

1 teaspoon chopped peanuts

1 teaspoon sesame oil

juice of ½ lime

½ red chilli, deseeded and chopped

sea salt and ground black pepper

Combine the shredded chicken, spinach, radishes, tomatoes, cucumber and peanuts on a serving dish.

Dress with the sesame oil, lime juice, chilli, salt and pepper. Serve warm or cold as a packed lunch.

Chicken Mint & Papaya Salad

125g (4½oz) cooked chicken breast, cubed

handful of mint leaves, chopped, plus extra leaves to garnish

½ handful of flat leaf parsley, chopped

½ cup chopped cucumber

½ large ripe papaya, cubed

1 tablespoon low-fat Greek yogurt

juice of ½ lime

sea salt and ground black pepper

lime zest, to garnish

Mix together the cubed chicken, half the mint leaves, the chopped parsley, cucumber and cubed papaya.

Make a dressing with the yogurt, lime juice, salt and pepper and the rest of the chopped mint. Drizzle over the salad and garnish with the whole mint leaves and lime zest.

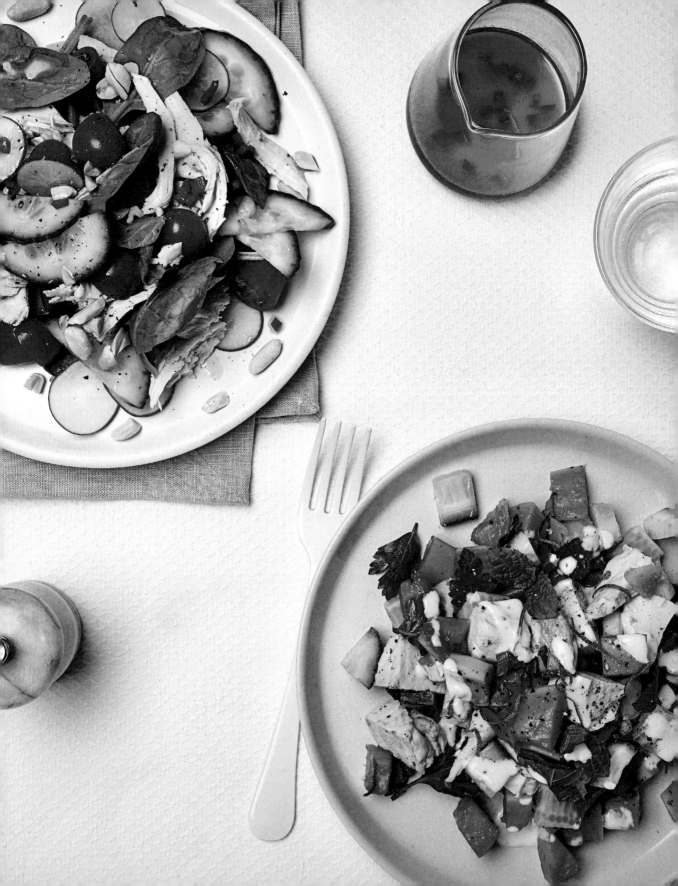

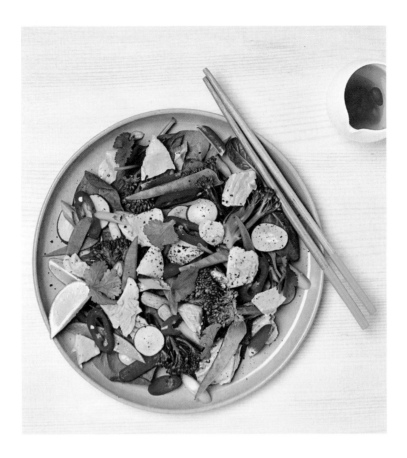

Asian Salmon Salad

5 handfuls of young leaf spinach

2 spring onions, chopped

2 radishes, sliced

1 cup cooked broccoli florets

1 cup blanched mangetout, sliced diagonally

½ red chilli, deseeded and sliced

75g (2¾oz) poached, grilled or
ready-cooked salmon fillet, flaked

2 teaspoons sesame oil

juice of ½ lime

sea salt and ground black pepper

coriander leaves, to garnish

Combine the spinach with the spring onions,
radishes, broccoli, mangetout and chilli.

Top with the flaked salmon, dress with the sesame
oil, lime juice and salt and pepper and garnish
with coriander leaves.

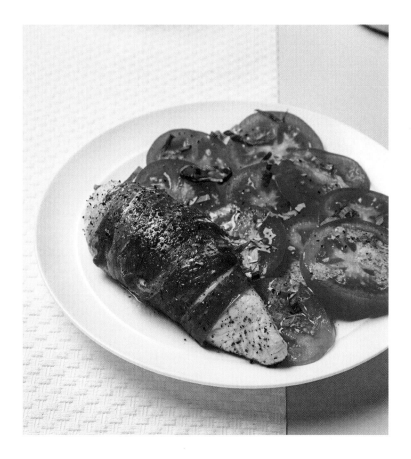

Prosciutto-wrapped Chicken with Tomato Basil Salad

125g (4½oz) chicken breast or mini chicken fillets

4 slices of lean prosciutto

2 beef tomatoes, sliced

few basil leaves, shredded

juice of ½ lemon

½ tablespoon olive oil

½ teaspoon Dijon mustard

sea salt and ground black pepper

Preheat the oven to 180°C (350°F), Gas Mark 4.

Wrap the chicken breast in the prosciutto slices, or wrap each mini chicken fillet in a single slice, and season with salt and pepper. Bake for about 15 minutes, until cooked through.

Serve with a tomato and basil salad, dressed with the lemon juice, olive oil, mustard and salt and pepper.

Antipasti Salad

4 slices of prosciutto

1 beef tomato, sliced

½ ball of buffalo mozzarella, sliced

12 large olives, pitted

2 artichoke hearts

handful of young leaf spinach and
rocket leaves

1 tablespoon balsamic vinegar

1 teaspoon reduced-fat pesto

sea salt and ground black pepper

Assemble the prosciutto with the
tomato, mozzarella, olives, artichokes
and spinach and rocket leaves.

Serve with a balsamic vinegar and
pesto dressing and season.

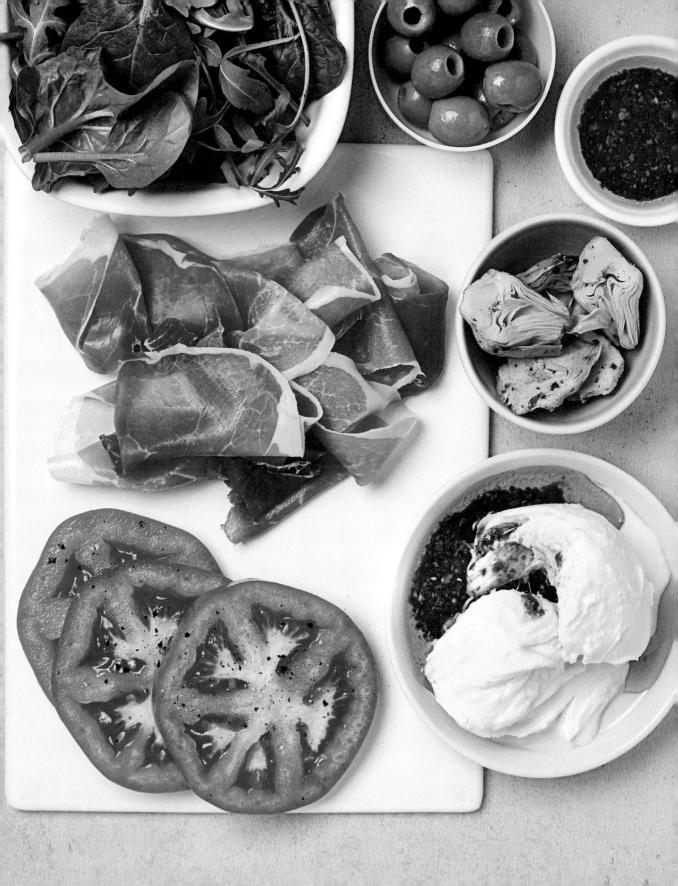

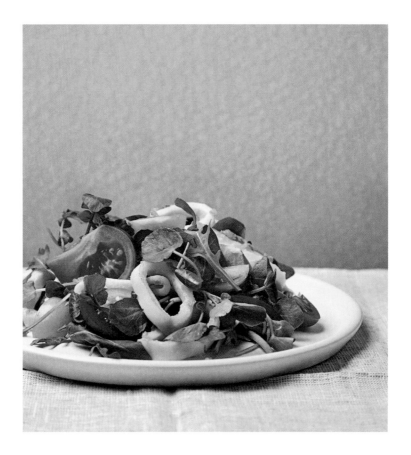

Chargrilled Squid & Salad

150g (5½oz) ready-cooked squid rings

handful of rocket and watercress leaves

8 heirloom tomatoes, halved and sliced

1 tablespoon low-fat Greek yogurt

juice of ½ lemon

½ teaspoon grated lemon zest

Arrange the squid rings on the salad of rocket, watercress and tomatoes. Dress with the yogurt, lemon juice and lemon zest.

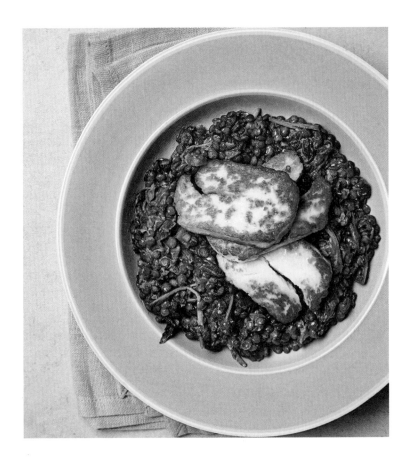

Puy Lentil & Haloumi Salad

1 teaspoon olive oil, for frying

¼ onion, ½ carrot and ½ celery stalk, diced

75g (2¾oz) Puy lentils

1 sprig of thyme

50ml (2fl oz) white wine

300ml (10fl oz) chicken stock

75g (2¾oz) spinach

1 teaspoon double cream

50g (1¾oz) haloumi cheese

sea salt and ground black pepper

Heat the olive oil in a frying pan over a medium heat and fry the onion, carrot and celery until soft. Wash and drain the lentils and add to the pan with the thyme and white wine.

Bring to the boil, add the stock, reduce to a simmer and cook for 30–35 minutes.

When the lentils are cooked, season well and add the spinach. Once the spinach has wilted, stir in the double cream.

In a separate pan, fry the haloumi with a little olive oil over a very high heat for 30 seconds on each side and serve on top of the lentils.

Spring Vegetable & Parmesan Frittata

Serves 4

1 tablespoon olive oil

1 red onion, finely diced

½ carrot, chopped

8 asparagus spears, chopped

¼ cup frozen peas

8 organic eggs

a little green chilli, deseeded and chopped (optional)

2 tablespoons grated Parmesan cheese

sea salt and ground black pepper

Heat the oil in a large omelette pan over a medium heat and stir-fry the onion, carrot, asparagus and peas until lightly cooked.

Beat the eggs really well and season with salt and pepper, and the chilli if using. Add the eggs to the pan and cook over a medium heat for 5 minutes until the bottom has browned nicely.

Sprinkle with the Parmesan, then pop under a medium grill for a further 5 minutes, or until the top has set and is turning golden.

Broad Bean, Pea & Bacon Salad

2 rashers of streaky bacon

2 handfuls of pea shoots or rocket

½ cup broad beans, lightly cooked and podded

½ cup peas, lightly cooked

10cm (4 inches) cucumber, sliced

2 spring onions, chopped

1 cup broccoli florets, blanched

1 teaspoon pesto

ground black pepper

juice of ½ lemon

Chop the bacon rashers and pan-fry until crispy.

Combine the pea shoots or rocket, broad beans, peas, cucumber, spring onions, broccoli and crisp bacon. Dress with the pesto, pepper and lemon juice.

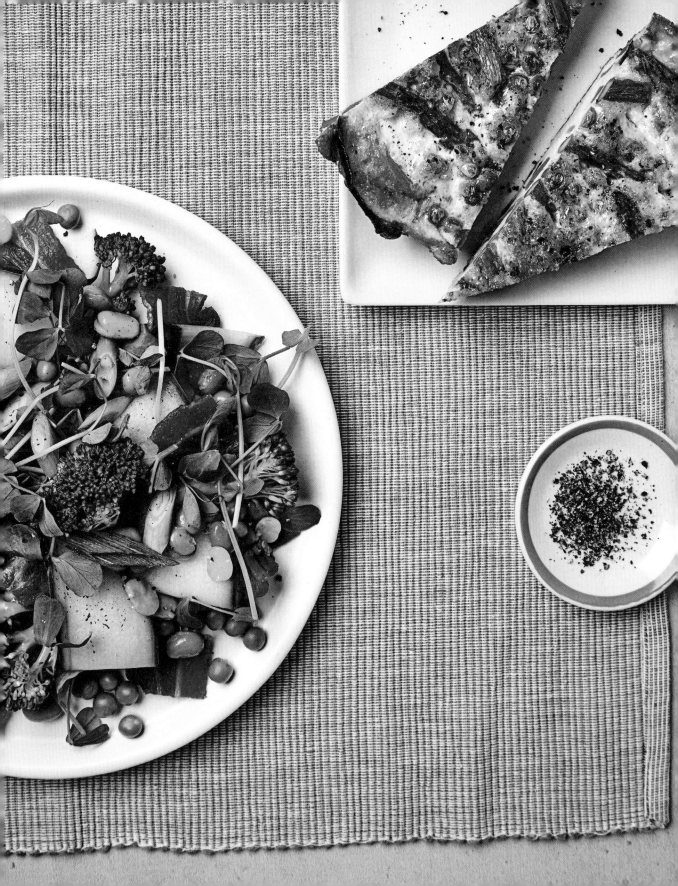

EVENIING MEALS

Savoy Eggs

2½ teaspoons olive oil

2 teaspoons mustard seeds

½ Savoy cabbage, very finely sliced

2 large organic eggs

½ red chilli, deseeded and sliced

1 tablespoon chopped flat leaf parsley, to garnish

sea salt and ground black pepper

Put 1 teaspoon of the olive oil and the mustard seeds in a wok and cook over a low heat with the lid on until the seeds pop. Remove from the wok and set aside.

Add 1 teaspoon of the olive oil, the cabbage and seasoning to the wok. Steam-fry (adding 1 tablespoon water every 3 minutes) for 6–9 minutes. Mix in the toasted mustard seeds and then set aside on a warmed plate.

Now fry the eggs in the remaining olive oil.

Serve the fried eggs on top of the cabbage, sprinkled with the chilli slices and garnished with parsley.

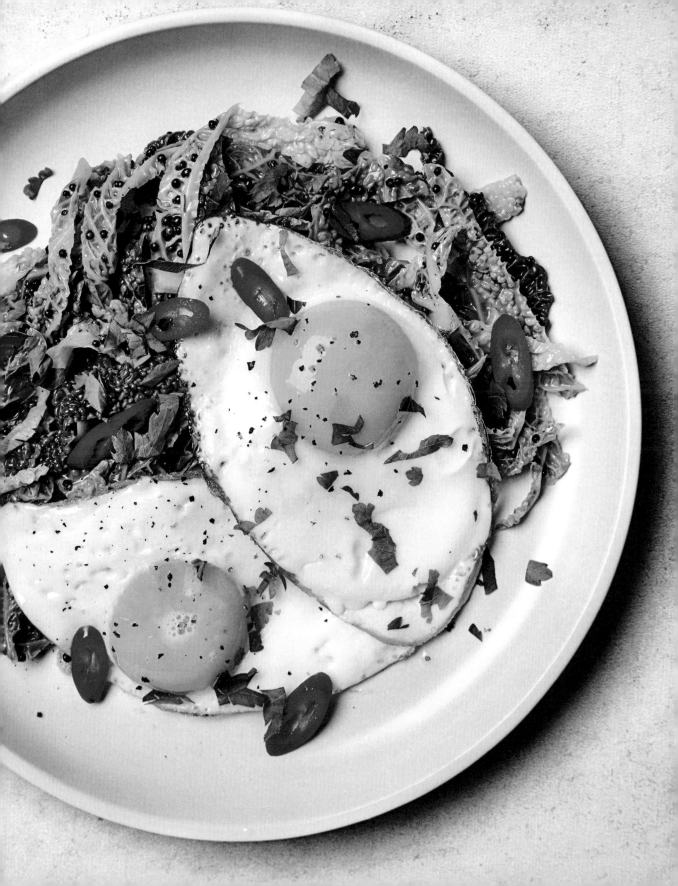

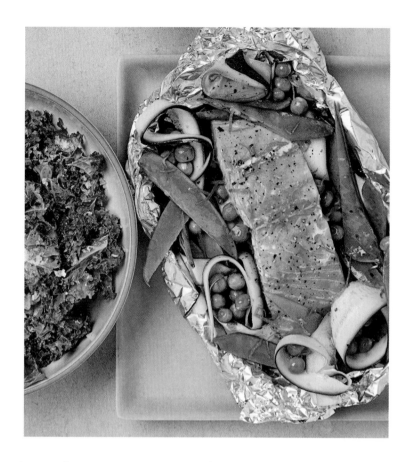

Federica's Salmon Parcels with Spring Vegetables

75g (2¾oz) salmon fillet

¼ cup frozen peas

4 baby courgettes, peeled into ribbons

1 cup mangetout, sliced diagonally

juice of ½ orange

½ teaspoon orange zest

2 tablespoons dry white wine

sea salt and ground black pepper

½ large bag of spinach or kale, wilted

Preheat the oven to 180°C (350°F), Gas Mark 4.

Wrap the salmon in a foil parcel, adding the peas, courgette ribbons, mangetout, orange juice and zest, white wine, salt and pepper. Bake for about 15–20 minutes, depending on how you like your salmon, then serve with the wilted spinach or kale.

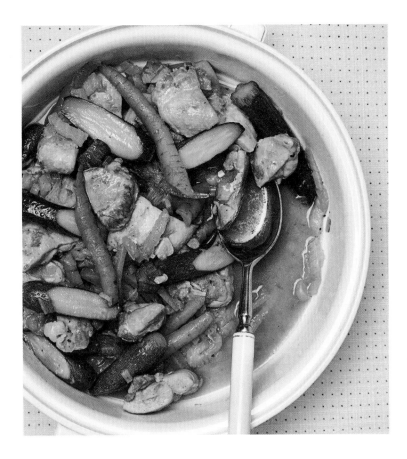

Sandi's Salvation Stew

1 tablespoon olive oil

2 shallots, chopped

½ fennel bulb, finely sliced

125g (4½oz) boneless chicken thighs, cut into quarters

2 garlic cloves, sliced

4 baby carrots, sliced in half diagonally

6 baby courgettes, sliced in half diagonally

50ml (2fl oz) good chicken stock

50ml (2fl oz) white wine

handful of tarragon leaves

1 portion of green vegetables, steamed (optional)

sea salt and ground black pepper

Preheat the oven to 180°C (350°F), Gas Mark 4.

Heat the olive oil in an ovenproof casserole and fry the shallots and fennel. Add the chicken thighs and cook over a high heat until the chicken is brown but not cooked through. Now add the garlic, carrots, courgettes, chicken stock, wine, tarragon leaves and seasoning.

Transfer the casserole to the oven and cook for 20–30 minutes until the chicken is tender. Serve with steamed green vegetables on the side, if liked.

Chicken, Chickpea & Chorizo Stew

1 small onion

25g (1oz) chorizo sausage

100g (3½oz) chicken thigh, skin removed and cut into quarters

¼ cup canned chickpeas

6 cherry tomatoes

½ yellow pepper, cored, deseeded and cubed

½ red pepper, cored, deseeded and cubed

½ cup chicken stock

chopped flat leaf parsley, to garnish

2 portions of green vegetables, steamed (optional)

Cube the onion and slice the chorizo, then pan-fry over a medium heat until the onion is translucent.

Add the chicken, chickpeas, tomatoes, yellow and red pepper and the chicken stock. Simmer over a low heat for 20 minutes, or until the chicken is cooked through, then garnish with chopped parsley.

Serve with the green vegetables on the side, if liked.

This recipe serves one, but is great to make in bulk and freeze.

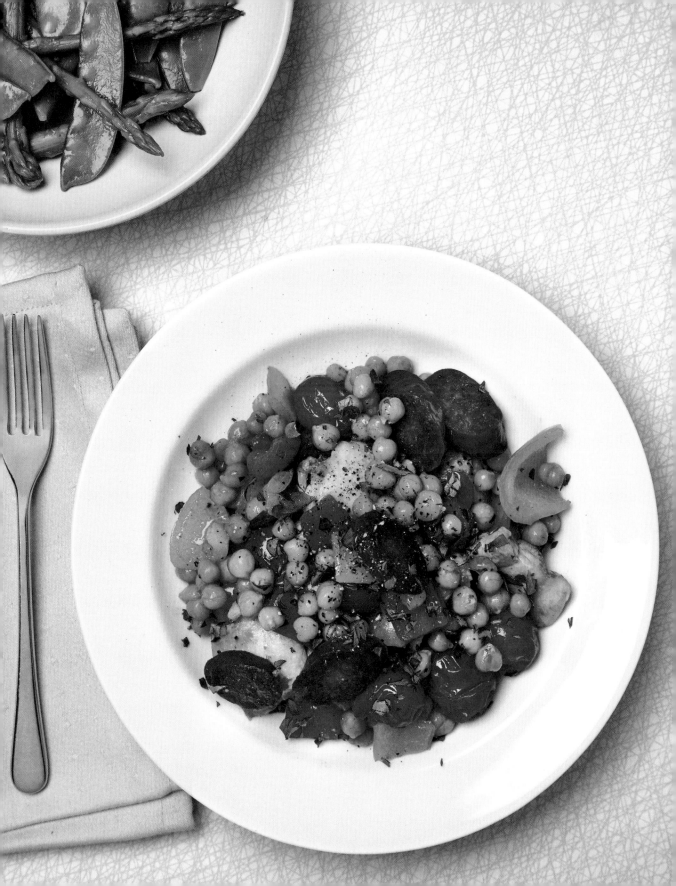

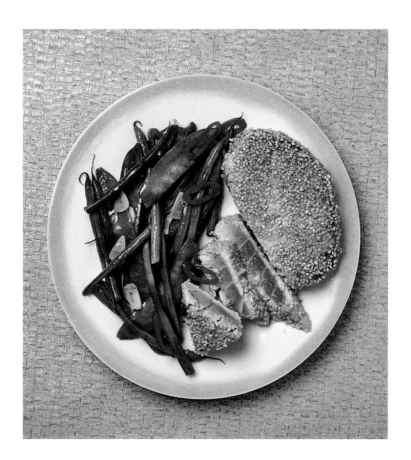

Sesame Tuna Steak
& Asian Vegetables

75g (2¾oz) fresh tuna steak

2 teaspoons groundnut oil

2 tablespoons sesame seeds

2 portions of green vegetables

2 teaspoons sesame oil

1 garlic clove, crushed

½ teaspoon chopped fresh ginger

2 teaspoons light soy sauce, or to taste

chopped coriander leaves, to garnish

Brush the tuna with half the oil then dip both sides in the sesame seeds. Pan-fry in the remaining oil over a medium heat, turning halfway, until golden.

Serve with green vegetables that have been steamed or stir-fried in the sesame oil, garlic and ginger. Add soy sauce to taste and garnish with coriander leaves.

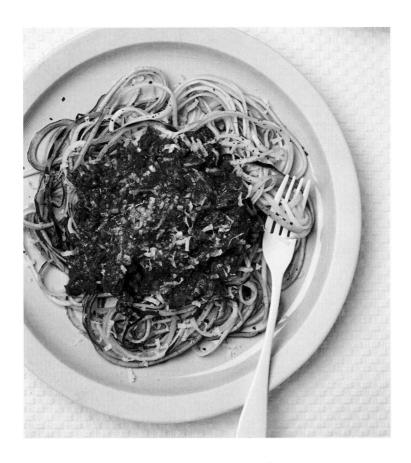

Courgetti Bolognese

1 tablespoon olive oil

2 onions, finely chopped

1 tablespoon dried herbes de Provence

800g (1lb 12oz) lean steak mince

700ml (1¼ pints) passata

1 × 400g (14oz) can cherry tomatoes

1 heaped tablespoon red pesto

¾ teaspoon ground black pepper

50ml (2fl oz) red wine

½ beef jelly stock cube

8 courgettes, spiralized

1 tablespoon grated Parmesan cheese

Serves 8

Preheat the oven to 150°C (300°F), Gas Mark 2.

Heat the oil in an ovenproof casserole and sweat the onions and herbs for 3 minutes over a low–medium heat. Add the mince and stir for 3 minutes until brown. Stri in the passata, tomatoes, pesto, pepper, red wine and beef stock. Transfer to the oven and cook slowly for 1½ hours, with the lid off, adjusting the seasoning to taste.

Serve the sauce on top of the raw spiralized courgettes, topped with Parmesan.

Smoked Tofu & Peanut Stir-fry

1 teaspoon sesame oil

1 garlic clove, crushed

a little fresh ginger, peeled and finely chopped

125g (4½oz) smoked tofu, diced

½ red pepper, cored, deseeded and sliced

2 spring onions, sliced

¼ cup soya beans

½ cup mangetout, sliced diagonally

1 cup bean sprouts

1 tablespoon reduced-salt soy sauce

1 teaspoon peanuts, toasted

Heat the sesame oil in a wok over a high heat and fry the garlic, ginger, tofu, red pepper, spring onions, soya beans, mangetout and bean sprouts for 2 minutes.

Add the soy sauce, then sprinkle with the toasted peanuts and serve immediately.

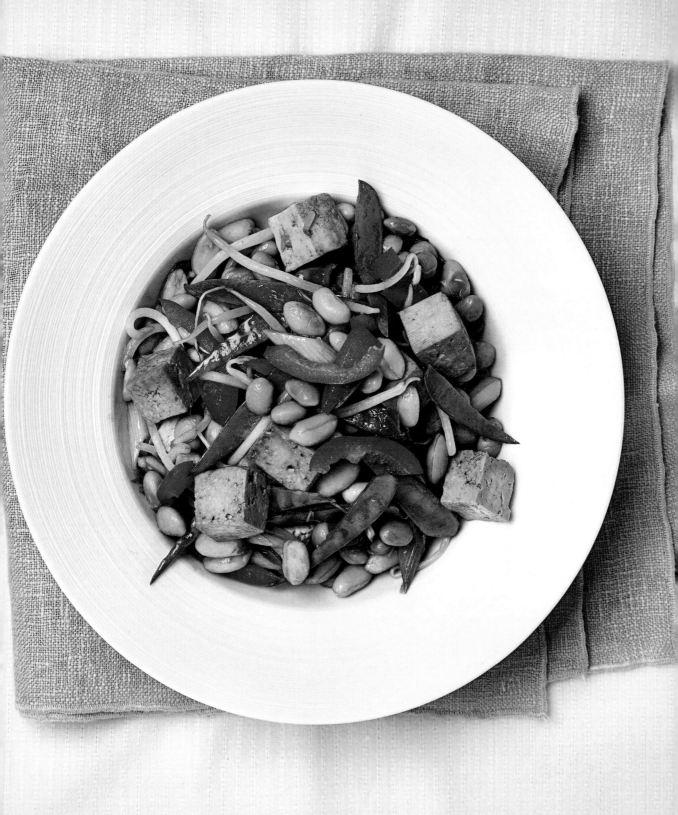

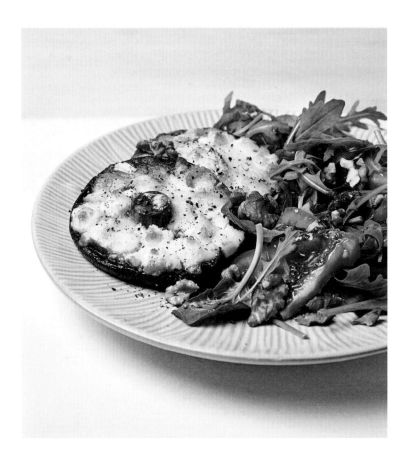

Grilled Goats' Cheese on Mushroom

1 large Portobello mushroom

olive oil, for spraying

75g (2¾oz) goats' cheese

handful of rocket and young leaf spinach

1 large beef tomato, sliced

1 tablespoon good balsamic vinegar

1 teaspoon reduced-fat pesto

6 walnuts, toasted and roughly chopped

Preheat the oven to 180°C (350°F), Gas Mark 4.

Spray the mushroom with a little oil, bake for 5 minutes, then remove from the oven. Preheat the grill.

Top the mushroom with the goats' cheese, and then cook under the grill for 2 minutes until the cheese starts to turn golden.

Serve with the rocket, spinach and tomato, dressed in balsamic vinegar and pesto and sprinkled with walnuts.

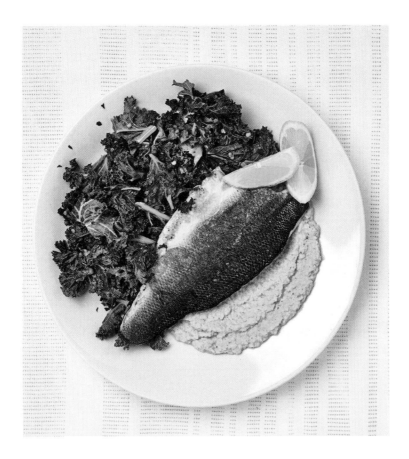

Lemon Sea Bass
with Vegetable Purée

150g (5½oz) sea bass fillet, skin on

1 teaspoon olive oil

juice of 1 lemon

2 cups of mixed frozen vegetables
(carrot, cauliflower, broccoli)

1 teaspoon butter

sea salt and ground black pepper

3 handfuls of kale, sautéed

1 teaspoon dried chilli flakes

lemon wedges, to garnish

Season the sea bass and pan-fry, skin side down, in the oil for 2–3 minutes until crispy. Turn carefully, add the lemon juice and cook for 1 minute more. Remove from the pan.

Steam the mixed vegetables until just cooked, then purée with the butter, adding salt and pepper to taste, until smooth.

Arrange the fish on top of the puréed veggies and serve with the sautéed kale, sprinkled with chilli flakes. Garnish with lemon wedges.

Scallops & Chorizo

25g (1oz) chorizo sausage

100g (3½oz) scallops

juice of ½ lemon

1 cos lettuce, chopped

5cm (2 inches) cucumber, halved, deseeded and sliced

12 sugarsnap peas, sliced diagonally

handful of flat leaf parsley, chopped

lemon wedges, to garnish

Gently fry the chorizo for 2 minutes in a dry, hot pan. Remove and set aside.

Now put the scallops in the pan and sear for 1 minute on each side.

Return the chorizo to the pan and squeeze over the lemon juice.

Combine the lettuce, cucumber, sugarsnap peas and parsley to make a salad.

Serve the scallops and chorizo on the salad and garnish with lemon wedges.

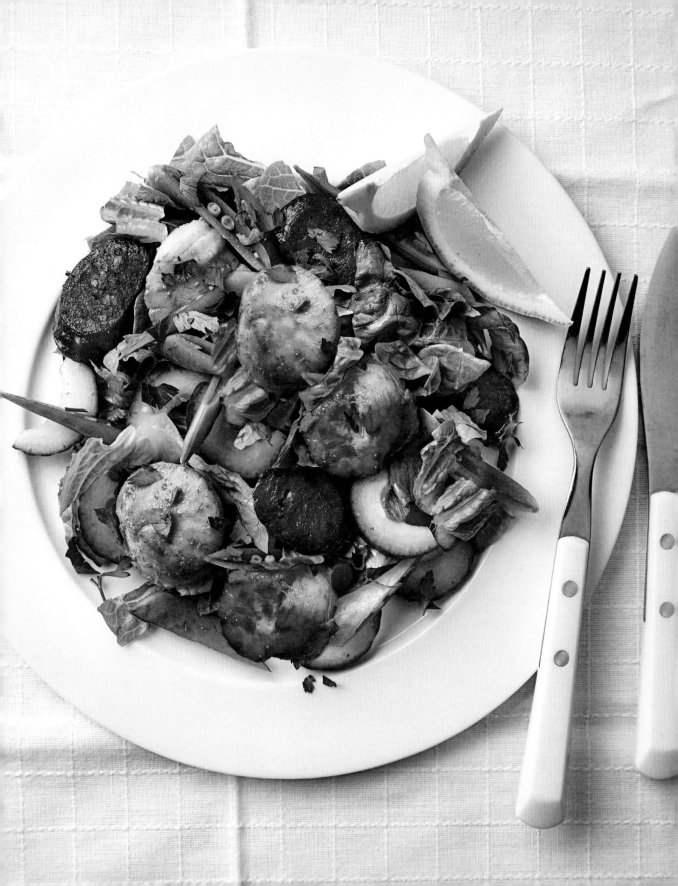

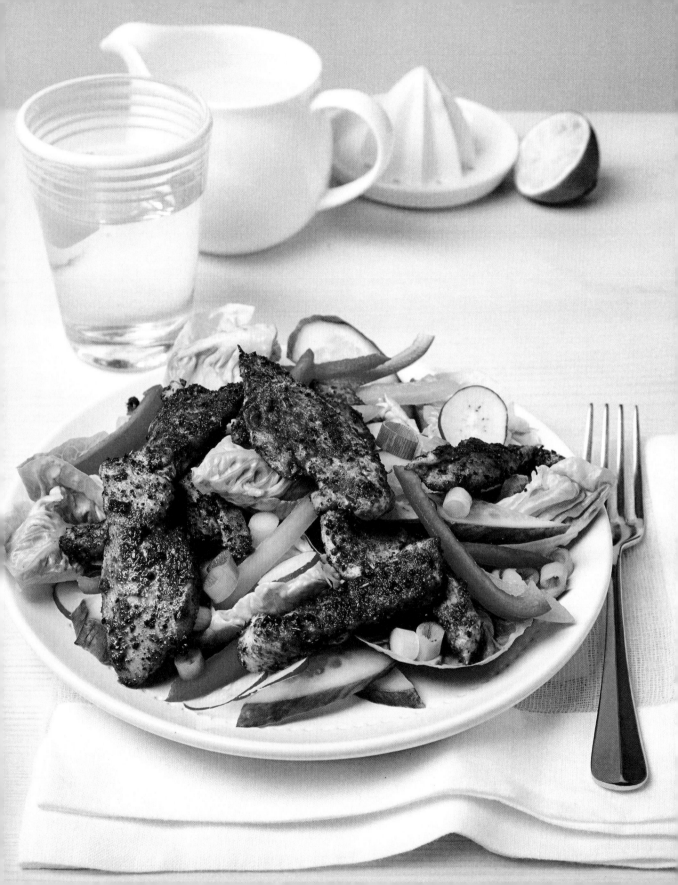

Cajun-spiced Chicken Salad

1 tablespoon Cajun spice mix

1 teaspoon olive oil

125g (4½oz) chicken breast, cut into strips

baby gem lettuce, leaves separated

7.5cm (3 inches) cucumber, sliced

4 radishes, sliced

½ red pepper, cored, deseeded and sliced

½ yellow pepper, cored, deseeded and sliced

2 spring onions, sliced

1 teaspoon olive oil

juice of ½ lime

Mix the Cajun spice with the olive oil, then rub all over the chicken strips. Fry over a medium heat for 15 minutes, or until cooked through.

Combine the lettuce, cucumber, radishes, peppers and spring onions to make a salad. Dress with the olive oil and lime juice.

Serve the Cajun-spiced chicken on the salad.

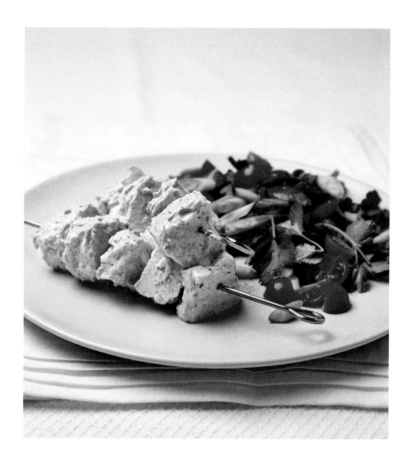

Pesto Chicken Kebabs

100g (3½oz) cooked chicken breast

50g (1¾oz) low-fat Greek yogurt

1 teaspoon green or red pesto

2 handfuls of coriander leaves

2 handfuls of flat leaf parsley

handful of mint

12 cherry tomatoes

1 spring onion

2 teaspoons olive oil

juice of ½ lemon

sea salt and ground black pepper

Cut the chicken breast into chunks and mix with the yogurt and pesto, then season to taste.

Finely chop the coriander, parsley, mint, tomatoes and spring onion. Dress the salad with the olive oil and lime juice, then season with the salt and pepper.

Skewer the chicken onto kebab sticks, if you wish, or simply serve it on the herby salad.

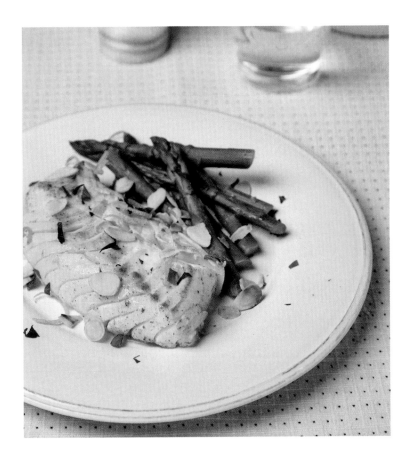

Almond Lemon Cod

150g (5½oz) cod fillet

1 teaspoon olive oil

1 teaspoon butter

juice of 1 lemon

1 tablespoon flaked almonds, toasted

chopped flat leaf parsley, to garnish

8 asparagus spears or any green
vegetable of your choice, steamed

sea salt and ground black pepper

Season the cod with salt and pepper and
pan-fry it in the olive oil and butter until golden
and crisp. Remove the cod from the pan, then
deglaze the pan with the lemon juice.

Pour the jus over the fish then top with the
toasted almonds and parsley. Serve with
the asparagus spears or green vegetable
of your choice.

Steak with Cauliflower Mash & Fennel

1 fennel bulb, quartered

1 teaspoon olive oil, plus extra for spraying

100g (3½oz) fillet steak

2 cups cauliflower florets, steamed

1 teaspoon butter

1 teaspoon fennel seeds

1 portion of green vegetables, steamed, to serve

sea salt and ground black pepper

Preheat the oven to 200°C (400°F), Gas Mark 6.

Cut the fennel into wedges, spray with the olive oil and roast for 30 minutes, or until golden.

Meanwhile, brush the steak with the 1 teaspoon olive oil, then season on both sides. Griddle over a high heat until cooked to your preference, and then leave to rest for 5 minutes.

While the steak is cooking and resting, mash the steamed cauliflower with the butter, sprinkle with fennel seeds and season to taste.

Slice the steak and serve it alongside the mash, roasted fennel and any green veggie you fancy.

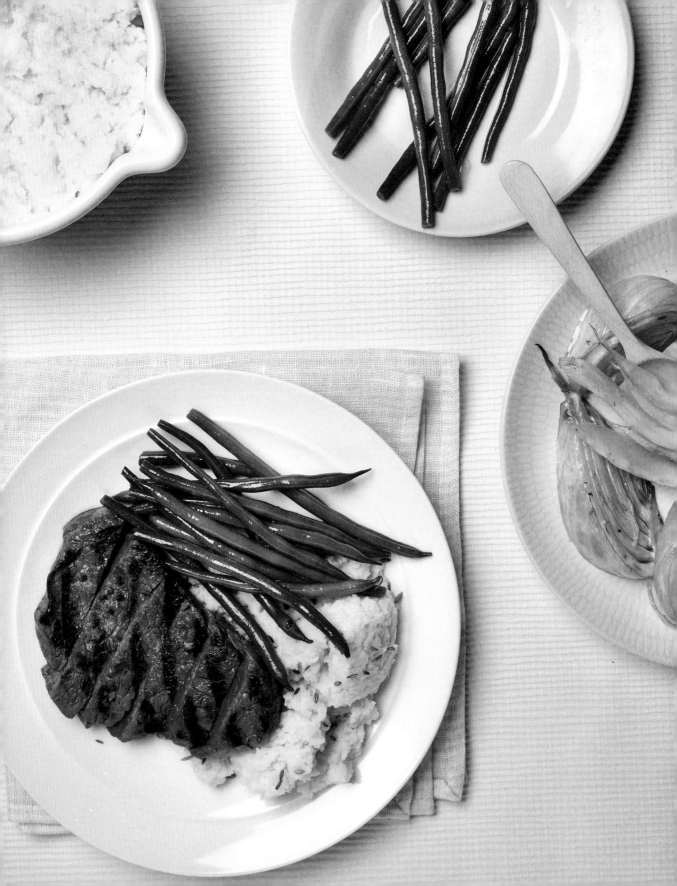

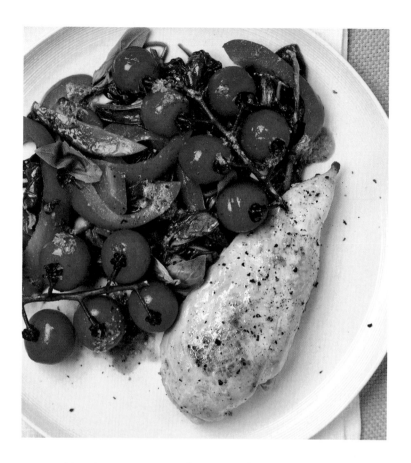

JT's Prada Chicken

125g (4½oz) chicken breast or lean thighs

12 cherry tomatoes on the vine

few basil leaves

1 teaspoon red or green pesto

1 red pepper, cored, deseeded and sliced

handful of spinach and mangetout

2 teaspoons olive oil

1 teaspoon good balsamic vinegar

sea salt and ground black pepper

Preheat the oven to 180°C (350°F), Gas Mark 4.

Secure the chicken, tomatoes, basil, pesto, red pepper, spinach and mangetout in a baking paper parcel. Bake for 20 minutes, or until the chicken is cooked through.

Season the chicken and herby veggies to taste and serve dressed with the olive oil and balsamic vinegar.

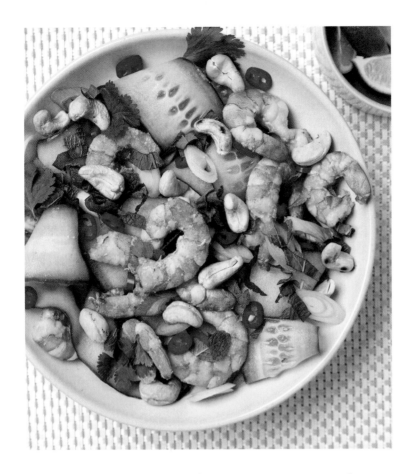

Prawn, Cucumber & Cashew Salad

1 teaspoon groundnut oil

125g (4½oz) king prawns, peeled and deveined

½ teaspoon chopped garlic

12cm (5 inches) cucumber, peeled into ribbons

handful each of coriander and mint leaves, chopped

½ red chilli, deseeded and sliced

1 spring onion, sliced

juice of ½ lime

¼ teaspoon stevia

2 teaspoons light soy sauce

1 tablespoon sesame oil

½ tablespoon cashew nuts, roasted and chopped

Heat the groundnut oil in a wok over a high heat and stir-fry the prawns for 4 minutes, adding the garlic for the last minute of the cooking time. Remove from the heat and set aside.

Place all the other ingredients, except the sesame oil and cashews, in the same wok and cook until al dente. Return the prawns to the wok and cook for 1 minute more.

Dress the salad with the sesame oil and scatter over the cashew nuts.

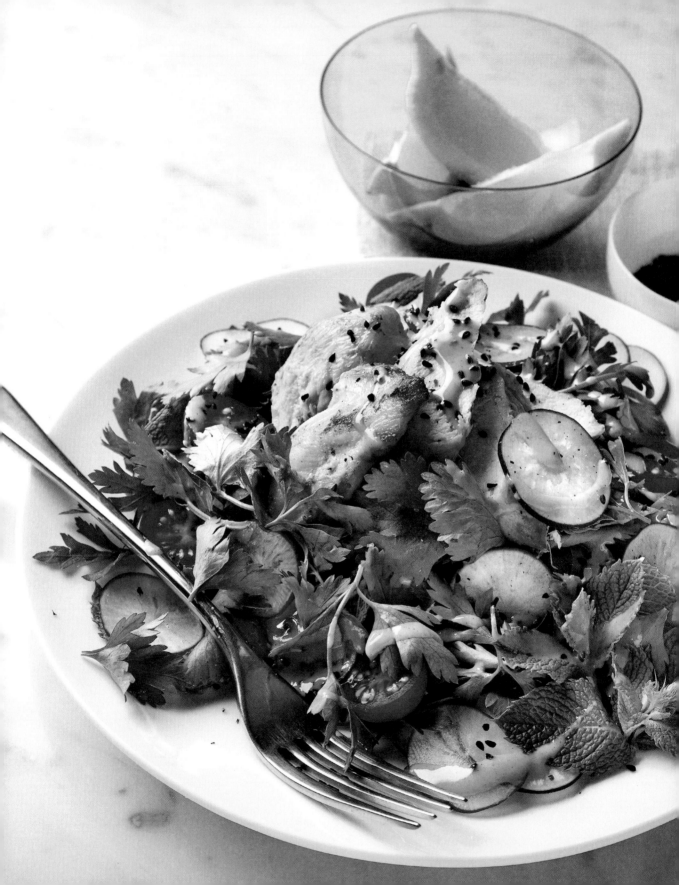

Marrakesh Salad

2 handfuls of coriander leaves

2 handfuls of flat leaf parsley

handful of mint

12 cherry tomatoes, halved

3 radishes, sliced

juice of ½ lemon

125g (4½oz) cooked chicken breast
(or 1 cup mixed beans or beluga lentils,
if you're vegetarian)

1 tablespoon tahini

1 teaspoon black onion seeds

sea salt and ground black pepper

few lemon wedges, to garnish

Finely chop the coriander, parsley and mint and add to a bowl. Add the tomatoes and radishes and season with the lemon juice and salt and pepper.

Slice the chicken breast and place it (or the pulses) on top of the other ingredients. Drizzle over the tahini and sprinkle with the black onion seeds. Serve with wedges of lemon.

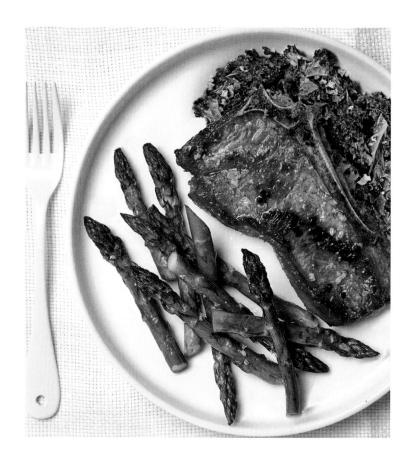

Veal with Mustard Butter & Asparagus

8 asparagus spears

2 sprays of olive oil

1 teaspoon Dijon mustard

2 teaspoons softened butter

100g (3½oz) veal steak

1 portion of green vegetables, steamed, or a mixed green salad, to serve (optional)

sea salt and ground black pepper

Preheat the oven to 180°C (350°F), Gas Mark 4.

Spray the asparagus with the olive oil and roast for 8 minutes.

Mix the mustard into the butter and season with salt and pepper. Spread the mustardy butter thinly on both sides of the veal steak and pan-fry for 5–6 minutes, turning halfway.

Serve the veal with the asparagus and add a steamed green veggie or a mixed green salad, if you like.

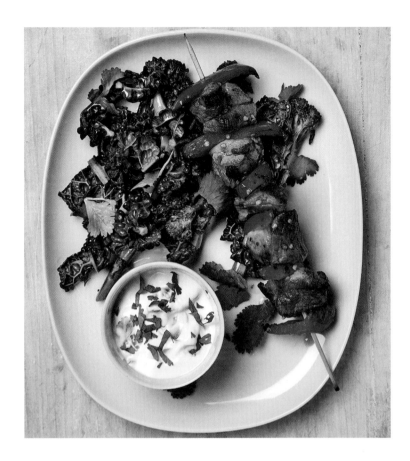

Lucy's Lithe Lamb

100g (3½oz) lean lamb, cubed

2 garlic cloves, crushed

juice of 1 lemon

1 teaspoon dried chilli flakes

1 red pepper, cored, deseeded and cut into chunks

2 tablespoons low-fat Greek yogurt

5cm (2 inches) cucumber, finely diced

coriander leaves or flat leaf parsley, roughly chopped, to garnish

sea salt and ground black pepper

2 portions of green vegetables, steamed

Marinate the lamb by securing it in a Ziploc bag with the garlic, lemon juice, chilli flakes and some salt and pepper for at least 1 hour, ideally overnight.

Preheat the grill to high. Thread the lamb onto a soaked skewer, alternating with chunks of red pepper. Place under the hot grill and cook, turning frequently, until the lamb is brown and tender.

Meanwhile, combine the yogurt and cucumber in a small bowl, season to taste and garnish with chopped coriander or parsley. Serve the kebabs alongside, accompanied by your choice of seasonal green vegetables.

Chicken Patties with Warm Pomegranate Slaw

125g (4½oz) chicken or turkey mince

1 spring onion, chopped

½ garlic clove, crushed

½ teaspoon grated lemon zest

½ teaspoon sea salt

½ teaspoon black pepper

½ tablespoon olive oil

Pomegranate slaw:

1 cup finely sliced Savoy cabbage

1 teaspoon groundnut oil

½ apple, halved, cored and sliced

juice of ½ lime

2 tablespoons pomegranate seeds

sea salt and ground black pepper

Mix the mince with the spring onion, crushed garlic, lemon zest, salt and pepper and then form the mixture into 2 patties. Heat the olive oil in a griddle pan over a medium heat and griddle the patties until golden and cooked through.

To make the slaw, stir-fry the cabbage over a high heat in the groundnut oil for 6 minutes, adding a tablespoon water every 2 minutes. Remove the cabbage from the heat and add the apple, lime juice and seasoning. Serve the chicken patties on the bed of warm slaw and sprinkle with pomegranate seeds.

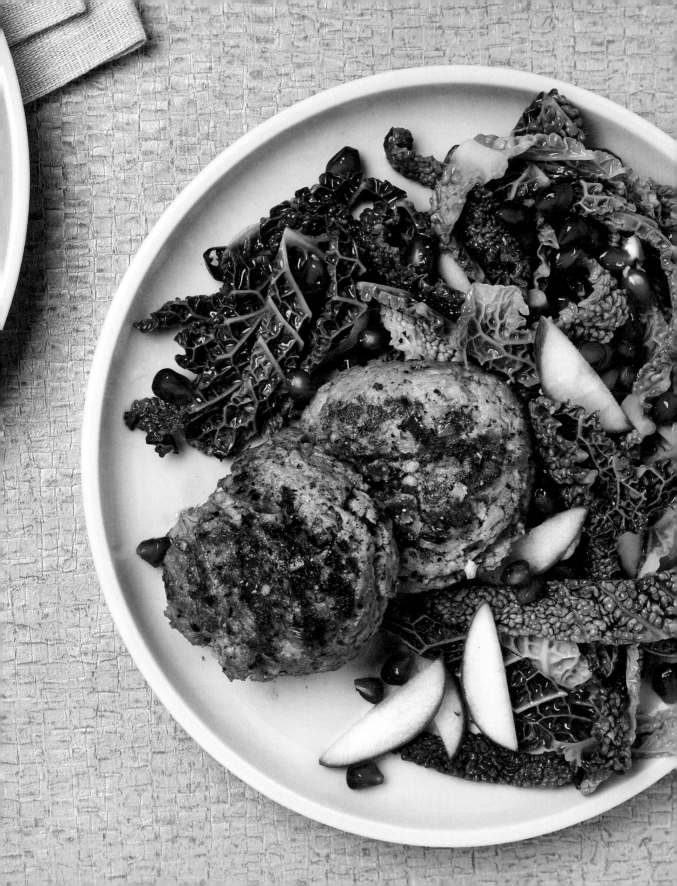

4

★ Weave activity into your everyday life, with an absolute minimum of 10,000 steps per day. Aim as high as you can

★ Complete a minimum of 15 minutes of my Louise Parker Method workout, which you can do at home with no kit

WORK OUT INTELLIGENTLY

With my Louise Parker workouts you'll achieve two things: a beautiful physical transformation, and the habit of exercise – just something you do every day, no matter what. Very simply, you'll move more. You're going to become someone who exercises every single day without having to rely on a gym, and we'll slot this into your life in the most efficient way possible.

The concise workouts with my favourite moves can all be done in the comfort of your own home. My Method is about getting you the most superb body and sustaining it with as little time and effort as you can get away with, so you're going to spend less time travelling and more time sculpting your body, without wasting a single minute.

Your home workouts consist of cardio-sculpting – so whilst you're raising your heart rate and burning fat, you're also going to be honing and toning your body, inch by inch. All the muscles in your body will be targeted: both the big ones that boost your muscle mass and metabolism, and the little muscles that sculpt you in the most elegant way.

Some of your workout days will be lighter, others more challenging, and you'll fit it all in around your mood and what else is going on in your life. I'll also teach you how to balance your workouts throughout the week.

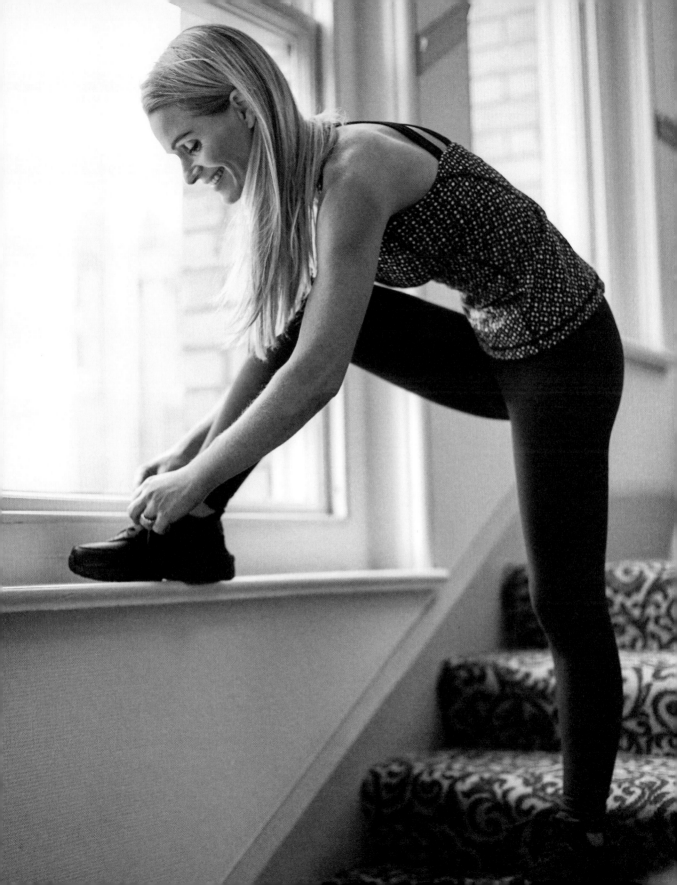

What Is a Louise Parker Body?

First, it has to be the body you want. I can't dictate to you
how lean or sculpted you should be. When you reach your
own visualization, you are there. But if you follow my
Method – all of it – you'll achieve a body that is lean and
tight. Every limb in your body will be sculpted and toned,
but in a delicate way. You won't have arms like a body
builder or thighs like a spinning instructor. You're going
to get a body that is elegant and more like that of a dancer.
The reason for this is that we are not going to overload it
with weight; we're going to overload it with repetition.
And the reason a dancer has such a beautiful body is
because they do reps, reps, reps – over and over again.
It's all about the reps.

Thirty per cent of our clients at Louise Parker are men –
and we use the same principle with them. They want to
have a sculpted, lean, strong body, but would rather look
like Brad Pitt with his shirt off than a bouncer. And the
reason Brad Pitt looks good with his shirt off is because
he does reps, reps, reps and doesn't train with very heavy
weights. So we use higher weights with men, but we
still don't do crazy weightlifting. That's not what we
are about at all.

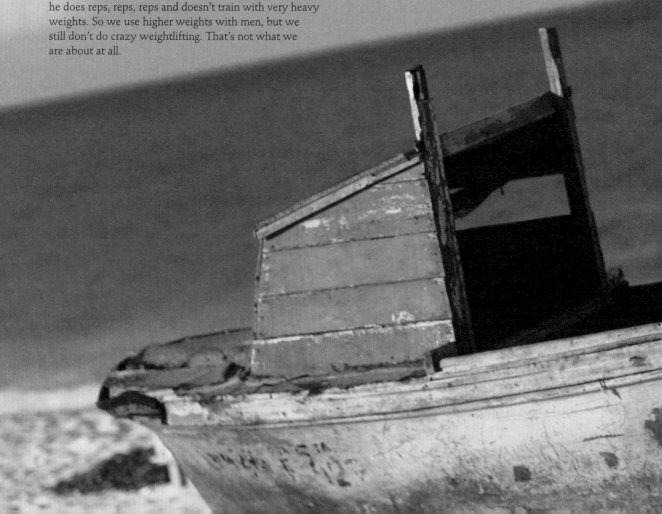

Energy In, Energy Out

Your body is burning energy all the time, even when you are sleeping. Your metabolism requires energy in the form of calories to support all the things that need to happen to keep you alive – building new cells, keeping that heart pumping, allowing your lungs to breathe in and out and to keep your body at a good temperature, among many other essential body processes. This is your basal metabolic rate (BMR), which you are going to boost through intelligently exercising, increasing your muscle mass and becoming more active. The higher your BMR, the more you're going to be able to eat and keep the fat off for good. So what you need to do is maximize the 'energy out', and my Method does this in the most time-efficient, practical way there is.

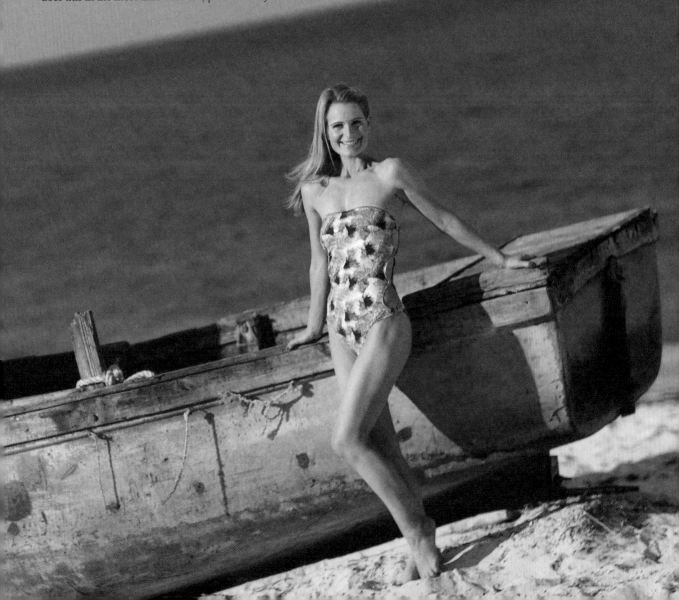

Be More Active

**This is where we start. We are meant to move.
Really, really move.**

I passionately believe that if you create the foundation of
being an active person, then the workouts you need to do
in order to be your best self are a million times more likely
to stick. **Your target should be at least 10,000 steps per
day**; buying a simple pedometer is a great way to track this.
This is the foundation on which my workouts are built.

Whilst my workouts are essential for you to achieve the
whole package, if you ignore the foundation – the being
active – then the effort required to stick to the habit of
your daily workout will always be greater. And I want
it to be as effortless as possible, so it lasts forever. Your
energy, motivation and drive will be greater when you
become an active person – so it's a critical foundation
of my Workout Method. Ignore this at your peril.

It's no good training three times a week, mentally ticking
the 'I work out' box, yet slobbing around the rest of the
time. This will not change your body, mindset or life.
We're meant to move, run, walk, play, and climb; we're not
designed to sit in cars or at desks all day and watch TV for
four hours a night. We have to get you moving and, as you
do, you will want to move more. It simply becomes a habit.
This habit will bring your body into beautiful balance when
you become an active person. Your skin will glow, your
hormones will behave and you'll feel happy, fit and free.

I don't want to patronize you with the 'Take the stairs'
chat, and I know we've all heard that a gazillion times.
It really irritates me when I read about doing your leg
exercises while you're waiting for the kettle to boil,
because I'm normally telling a child to use a plate and
trying to remember if it's ballet or gymnastics today.
But you know what: it is smart to find ways of sneaking
in exercise, and we'll do it in a way that isn't ridiculous.
I'm going to give you good, practical ideas on how you
can get more movement into your every day life.

I have a handful of clients who train 90 minutes a day
with my team, six days a week, and spend the rest of their
time staring at a trading screen that they simply cannot
leave. They're driven home, eat and go to bed, then repeat
the cycle the next day. So these sessions are essential to
prevent them dying of inactivity and stress, because they
literally do not move for the other 22½ hours a day. Most
of us don't have access to daily personal training, but
neither do we have to sit still all the time. We have the
opportunity to move – or at least I hope you do.

I'm in the habit of being active. I literally cannot sit and
work for a five-hour stretch at a time, like some of my
friends do. When I was writing this book I set the timer
on my phone and worked for 45 minutes, then got up,
grabbed a drink and did a few minutes of exercise. If I
don't do that, my body feels stiff, my brain stops working
and I just feel out of sorts. I'll do 50 walking lunges down
my hall, or do a few squats with CoCo. The point is: you
need to get up and move at least every 45 minutes. Even if
it's a walk up and down the stairs to grab yourself a drink.

If you work in an office, set your timer to remind you
to get up every 45 minutes. Pop out to the shops for a
bottle of water. Or walk eight flights of stairs. Don't lose
your job, but if the smokers are allowed out, then you
should be able to do some stair-walking. At lunchtime
walk for 30 minutes. Walk home or at least part walk
home. An actress I know turns her music up and cleans
and vacuums like Beyoncé, despite the fact that she
could afford an army of staff – she enjoys it, and it
keeps her fit and grounded.

Just put energy and oomph behind everything you do.
If you're a mum at home, vow to dance like no one is
watching, to three full tracks, before you tackle your day.
You'll be in a far better mood, I promise. After school
pick-up, take the kids to the park and really play: make
them scoot with you, whilst you power-walk or jog. Take
the bikes out around the park, hire a pedalo, go for family
walks and play Poohsticks; treat yourself to rollerblades
and have fun playing. Your children – and your backside –
will thank you for it for years to come.

I can't believe I'm saying this, but wear shoes you're
likely to walk in. I have a Manolo addiction and, on my
office days, I notice that I walk around far less. When I
leave the office I wear shoes I can walk in, to tempt me
out of a cab, and I'll walk home with a glow on and an
extra £8 in my pocket. On days when I've got my Nikes
on, I'm scooting about like the Duracell bunny – I feel
more bouncy, get more done and turn into an active me.

You have to weave activity into your lifestyle and stop
thinking about it as driving to the gym three times a
week. I'm no gym-bunny, and so whilst this all sounds
a bit goody-goody fitness talk, I promise that it's the
easy route. By weaving more activity into your lifestyle,
you can spend less time driving to the gym and walking
on a treadmill – which has to be the most life-zapping
exercise there is.

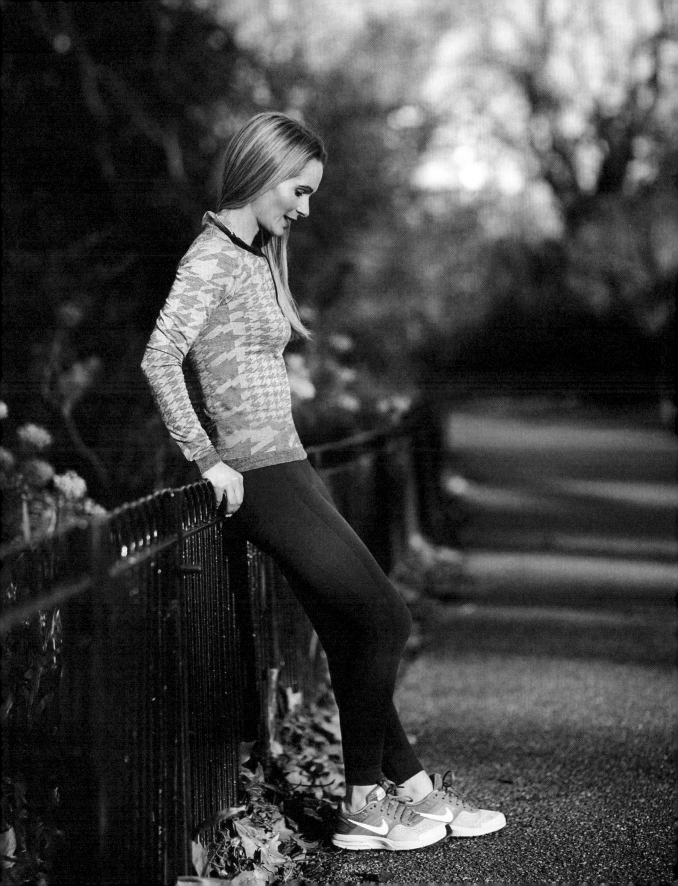

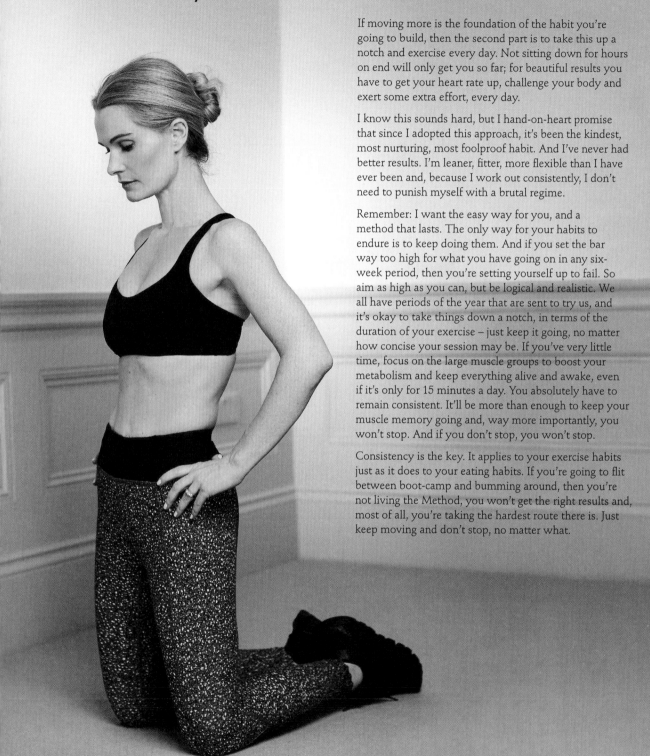

Move Daily, No Matter What

If moving more is the foundation of the habit you're going to build, then the second part is to take this up a notch and exercise every day. Not sitting down for hours on end will only get you so far; for beautiful results you have to get your heart rate up, challenge your body and exert some extra effort, every day.

I know this sounds hard, but I hand-on-heart promise that since I adopted this approach, it's been the kindest, most nurturing, most foolproof habit. And I've never had better results. I'm leaner, fitter, more flexible than I have ever been and, because I work out consistently, I don't need to punish myself with a brutal regime.

Remember: I want the easy way for you, and a method that lasts. The only way for your habits to endure is to keep doing them. And if you set the bar way too high for what you have going on in any six-week period, then you're setting yourself up to fail. So aim as high as you can, but be logical and realistic. We all have periods of the year that are sent to try us, and it's okay to take things down a notch, in terms of the duration of your exercise – just keep it going, no matter how concise your session may be. If you've very little time, focus on the large muscle groups to boost your metabolism and keep everything alive and awake, even if it's only for 15 minutes a day. You absolutely have to remain consistent. It'll be more than enough to keep your muscle memory going and, way more importantly, you won't stop. And if you don't stop, you won't stop.

Consistency is the key. It applies to your exercise habits just as it does to your eating habits. If you're going to flit between boot-camp and bumming around, then you're not living the Method, you won't get the right results and, most of all, you're taking the hardest route there is. Just keep moving and don't stop, no matter what.

Find a Way

You have to be accountable to yourself and find a way to be more active. I can't physically do this for you, and I've given you some ideas, but you have to truly take on board how you can make some changes. You have to do the work, the planning – you're responsible for that.

Whatever obstacles you have, which you think prevent you from being more active, write them down. Now look at them and force yourself to come up with a solution that will overcome them. If you think there isn't an obstacle, then you're lying to yourself, doing yourself a disservice and not letting me help you. You have to find ways of building more movement into your life, and it's possible for everyone.

Okay, here's where I shame you into it (sorry, but not sorry).

I used to live on Wimbledon Common and I'd just had my first daughter, Sophie, and was struggling with what I now think was post-natal depression, and my motivation was very low. There was this man – if you live in Wimbledon you'll know who I mean, because everyone in Wimbledon knows this man. He has one leg. Rain or shine, he is out running. Yes, running. With two sticks, hurling himself from one stride to another, without a prosthetic leg. And at a furious pace, no T-shirt on, sweat dripping from his ripped chest. I'd like to say he was my light-bulb moment to get me off my Pity Pot, and that I took up long-distance running the very next day, but I'd be lying. But perhaps, after I saw him a dozen times, I put on my Nikes and started power-walking off the baby fat – every single day, rain or shine. If he could do it with one leg, I could damn well do it with two. We have to learn to move and work around every niggle, injury or challenge we have.

My personal challenge is that I have acute chronic pain. I have this muscle in my upper back that is in constant spasm and I've had it for more than a decade, following two accidents that I had six weeks apart. It hurts if I rest it, it hurts if I train – so I just train and, over time, I have learned to live with this pain. There have been months when I've not trained, hoping for it to get better; but, honestly, using it as an excuse. There are days that are very hard and nights when I do not sleep, but I will not let this pain be bigger than I am. Sometimes I imagine that it is this power inside me, fuelling me to be the best I possibly can be. I don't talk about it much, because when I talk about it I think I feed the pain, and not the solution. I'd rather be in pain and in the best physical shape I can than in pain, overweight and living on the Pity Pot. You have to see the obstacle and step right over it.

So whether your obstacle is time, pain, disability, negativity, depression or addiction, acknowledge what it is and find a way round it. When you do, you will awaken the brilliance within you.

You have to see the obstacle and step right over it. When you do, you will awaken the brilliance within you

The Louise Parker Workouts

Dynamic from Day One

Everything you do in your workouts is going to focus on pace, energy and passion. We're going to prepare you for your workouts with dynamic stretching. This is a stretch that's performed through actual exercises – so you're essentially going straight into your workout, and stretching and mobilizing your body at the same time. It's going to improve your function, loosen your joints, warm up your body beautifully and prevent injury.

Maximize Every Minute

We're going to maximize the return on your time investment and not waste a precious minute. We'll move from one exercise to another at pace and won't waste time resting between sets. When you're resting one muscle, you're working another. We're going to multitask your muscle work so that you can spend less time training and more time getting on with life.

Simultaneous Sculpting

Then we will sculpt multiple muscles in each exercise, in a series of circuits, so that you get the job done faster, keep your heart rate up and your fat-burning tap dripping like crazy. We won't work your biceps and then rest, then do squats and rest. The more muscles you are working simultaneously, the more your mind is going to connect with your body, and this will feel amazing and will make time fly.

All-in-one Cardio-sculpting

Because you're working so many muscles at once in a constant flow of movement with high repetitions, your heart rate is going to be elevated. It will need lots of energy to keep up, and this energy is going to come from fat storage.

So with the reps, the dynamic pace and the multiple muscles firing at once, your heart rate is going to be really up. You're actually doing cardio whilst you are sculpting – you're getting the fat-burning benefits of a jog whilst you're toning your body: getting two jobs done at once. No more wasting time on the treadmill, zoning out. You're going to zone in and lean out.

Fat-burning Tap in Full Flow, 24 Hours a Day

Because we've challenged your muscles and heart rate, your body is going to switch to an impressive 'afterburn effect' (EPOC or 'excess post-exercise oxygen consumption', to get technical). I've been preaching for years that it's not all about the calories you burn *during* your workout; it's about the calories you burn *after* the session.

When you train you essentially damage your muscle fibres, in a good way, and then burn extra calories as you repair and rebuild them. As you build more muscle, you burn more calories both at rest and when you are training. It's why counting how many calories you burned on your exercise bike is a total waste of time.

You're Going to Progress

We're slowly going to build up the intensity of your workouts. If you're starting out not at your strongest, you'll go at a slower pace and do shorter workouts. But you'll be astounded by how fast you improve, and soon you'll be doing triple what you did in your first session. It's important that you do progress, because there's an immense link between the number of calories your body is going to burn after an intense session and the duration of your workout.

For most of us, the 'afterburn' is going to mean turning up that fat-burning tap when your heart rate is between 70 and 85 per cent of the maximum heart rate in your workout session. You can use a heart-rate monitor, but I prefer to make sure that I'm working to at least an 8/10 effort. You know when you're working hard or not – and you don't need to put in your greatest session every day: you're human and you're going to have days when you just get a little something done. You're simply going to do your best every day.

We're going to combine working your large muscles and the smaller, more delicate muscles in each and every session. This is going to give your body the most beautiful form and function, because all 600 muscles in your body are going to be engaged. We're going to train them six

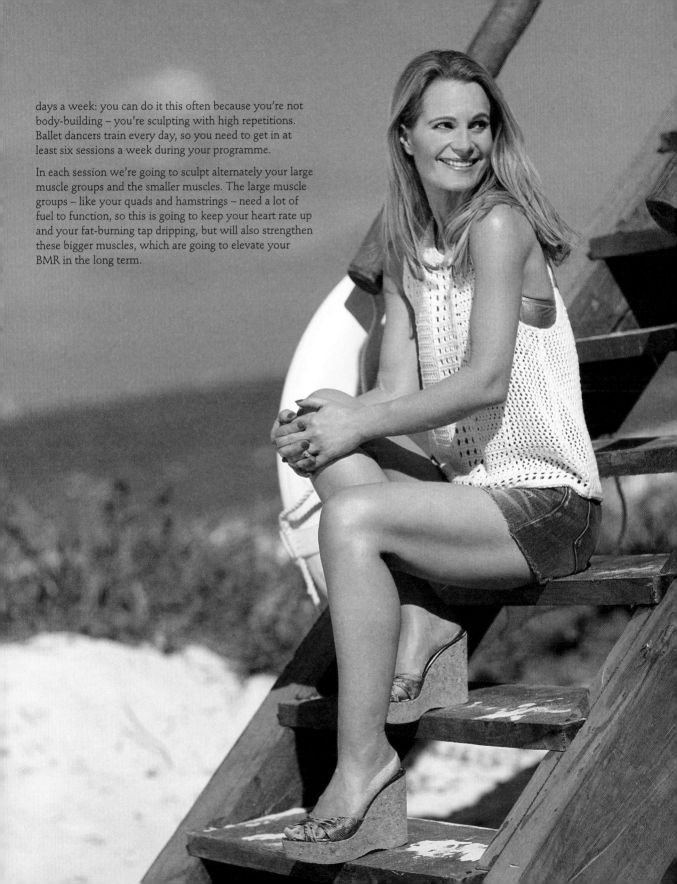

days a week: you can do it this often because you're not body-building – you're sculpting with high repetitions. Ballet dancers train every day, so you need to get in at least six sessions a week during your programme.

In each session we're going to sculpt alternately your large muscle groups and the smaller muscles. The large muscle groups – like your quads and hamstrings – need a lot of fuel to function, so this is going to keep your heart rate up and your fat-burning tap dripping, but will also strengthen these bigger muscles, which are going to elevate your BMR in the long term.

It's Not My Way OR the Highway

I obviously believe that the Louise Parker Method of training is going to yield you the very best results in the most time-efficient and sustainable way – or I'd have thought of something else over the last 20 years. However, I don't believe that it's a case of 'My way *or* the highway'.

I do want you to do my routines six days a week as a minimum, because I want you to tone and shred fat as swiftly as possible. And in terms of time-efficiency and results, you're going to get the best bang for your buck – workouts that are practical, and results and habits that last.

However, if you already do a barre class, or catch up with your best friend at Pilates, or love to go for a run at the weekend, don't drop it. Ultimately I want you moving more forever, so if there's a routine in place that you adore, keep doing it.

There are just a few things to be aware of:

Get Your Glow On

In addition to a minimum of 10,000 steps a day, you're going to be doing your workouts – as often as you can. You have to get a sweat on. You don't have to be dripping and huffing and puffing, but you must get a glow on and feel that your heart rate is up. If any of your regular workouts aren't challenging you in this way, or you don't feel your muscles working and engaging, it's time to move up to a more advanced class. You know if you're coasting – and, if you are, you have to take things up a notch.

Reduce Your Cardio and HIIT it

Yes, you need cardiovascular exercise, and I am not anti-cardio at all. What I passionately don't want you doing is primarily cardio work and ignoring all your conditioning workouts – because then you will never get the toned body you are after. I'm assuming you're reading my book because you want the most time-effective way of sculpting your body, burning fat and boosting your metabolism so that you can keep the fat off for ever. My workouts sculpt you and keep your heart rate up, so we're going to do cardio-conditioning and kill two birds with one stone.

If you're doing pure cardio as one or many of your weekly workouts – spinning, running, jogging, power-walking, swimming (of course these all tone muscles too, but not in the same way as my workouts), then I urge you to reduce them – in both quantity and duration. And you simply have to add in my strength and conditioning workouts or you'll end up 'skinny fat' – and that's not at all what we are after.

So if you're currently jogging for 40 minutes three times a week, drop it to one or two sessions and add in four of my workouts. Now reduce the duration of your jog to half the time and undulate the intensity, for maximum afterburn. Instead of plodding for 40 minutes, you're better off doing interval training for half the time. HIIT (High-Intensity Interval Training) means simply undulating your heart rate. So, if you're a beginner, you could do a lap around the park for 20 minutes (jogging for two minutes, running for one, sprinting for one and then walking, and repeat). There are endless combinations, and don't get hung up on the ratios. But make sure that when you are doing cardio, you are undulating: taking your heart rate up to that high point, back down, then back up again – you get the idea. If you're not getting a glow on, you're not doing it right.

The More You Give, the More You Get

Do the *very best* you can every single day – both throughout your programme and for ever. It's no use mumbling, 'I'm doing my best' – you have to take the biggest step you can every day, towards what is necessary for you to succeed. Some days are going to really test you; do a 15-minute circuit anyway. Force yourself and hold yourself accountable.

The next day you'll feel brighter and may do the routine two or three times. Just don't stop. Be under no illusions that if you want eye-watering, staggering results, you have to put in more than 15 minutes three times a week. However, if that is truly all you can do, do it – and put every single ounce of energy behind each movement. Make it count. If you half-arse it, you are going to get a half-arsed result. And I would like you to have a very nice arse.

Every single good thing in life worth possessing – a child, a career, your relationships, your faith, your precious body – requires strokes of daily effort. Lord knows, some days it's all I can do to get through my meetings and put my kids to bed alive. But on other days you have to dance a little harder, practise like you're on *Strictly* – and in the end the balance will work out. You have to pay your daily rent to success.

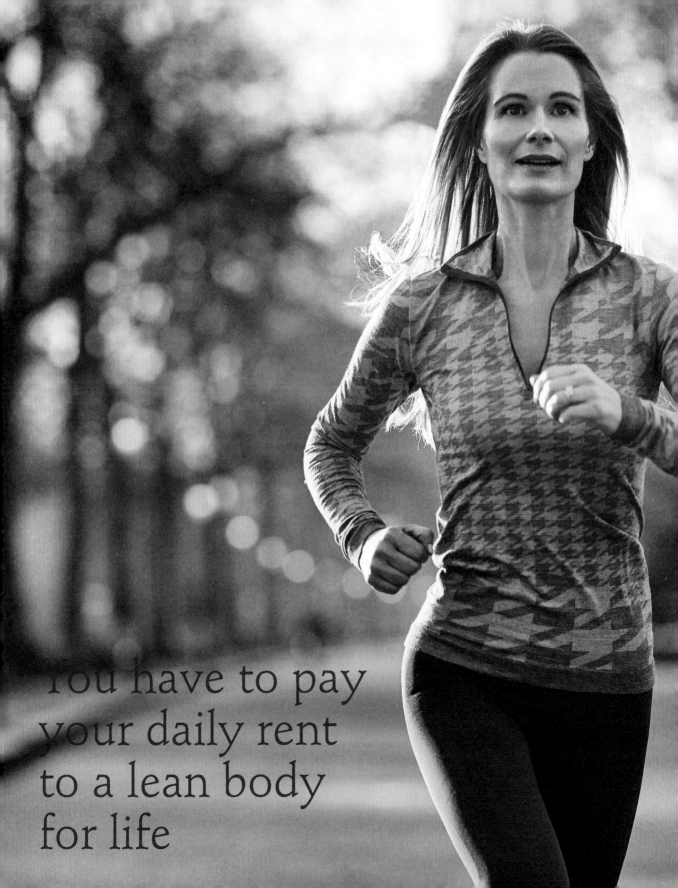

You have to pay
your daily rent
to a lean body
for life

The Workouts

I've chosen 20 of my absolute favourite exercises that will combine beautifully to burn fat, sculpt your body slim and tighten every delicate muscle in your body. Best of all, they can be performed at home, with absolutely no equipment at all.

Your routine will take a minimum of 15 minutes a day, after a short but non-negotiable warm-up lasting less than 5 minutes. Your body is going to adapt super-fast and soon you'll be ready to double and triple the length of your workouts, for even more eye-watering results.

I want you to do this at least six times a week – no matter what. Even if you've had the day from hell and you're bleeding from the eyeballs with tiredness, do *something* – even if you have to cut the routine down to 10 minutes of moves whilst your bath is running. I promise that this is the key to changing your workout habits for life. On days when I want to weep with exhaustion, I may just do eight minutes whilst the bath is filling with something glorious and relaxing. And I always, always feel better for it. Remember: if you don't stop, you won't stop. Just keep it moving.

I've split the exercises into two groups. The 'Classics' (see page 174) generally challenge your bigger muscle groups – the ones that really get your heart rate up and your fat-burning tap dripping, and they strengthen those larger muscles that will elevate your BMR (see page 153) long-term. The 'Sculpt' Exercises (see page 186) are generally a little more elegant – they remain focused on the large muscle groups, but bring into play the smaller muscles that are going to really sculpt you in the most elegant way possible. They will all build 'non-bulky' muscles, burn fat and sculpt you in the most sensational way.

For each daily workout, simply pick two 'Classics' and two 'Sculpt' moves. You'll complete each exercise for one minute, and then swap swiftly to the next exercise, alternating between Classic and Sculpt moves. Each four-exercise circuit will take approximately five minutes to complete (allowing you time to move between them) and you repeat this three times for your 15-minute workout. Use the stopwatch on your phone or a clock to help you manage the timings of your sessions.

A 15-minute workout looks like this:

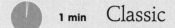 1 min Classic

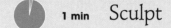 1 min Sculpt

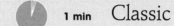 1 min Classic

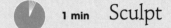 1 min Sculpt

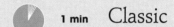 1 min Classic

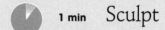 1 min Sculpt

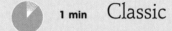 1 min Classic

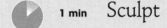 1 min Sculpt

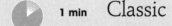 1 min Classic

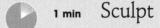 1 min Sculpt

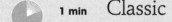 1 min Classic

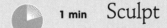 1 min Sculpt

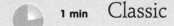 1 min Classic

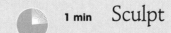 1 min Sculpt

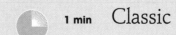 1 min Classic

How Do I Pick My Exercises Each Day?

There is no 'right order' in which to complete the exercises, so don't worry about this too much. I'd actually like you to pick your exercises randomly, so that you're always getting a varied workout – just put a tick beside the ones that you've done, so that you know which exercises you've been doing more of and which you've been avoiding. We tend to gravitate towards the moves that we love because we're good at them, so consider doing more of the ones that challenge you, both mentally and physically. This is something that I have to be constantly aware of – and it's an important part of creating and maintaining a functional, balanced body.

How Long Are My Workouts?

You're going to aim to do a minimum of the 15-minute routine most days (20 minutes including the warm-up). I know that even the most time-starved people can do this – I've seen it and coached it a zillion times. We're all busy, but remember: you're going to make it happen, no matter what. We're bringing you back to the top of the pile.

I'd love you to do this six days a week, and to increase the duration as soon as your body tells you it's ready. You'll just know. I promise, in a couple of weeks you'll be able to do the 15-minute routine twice – and then three times, in another fortnight.

If the most time you can initially dedicate is 20 minutes a day, then by Weeks Three and Four you should be aiming to increase this to 30 minutes, and then again in Weeks Five and Six.

But on time-starved days, just do what you can. As long as you are genuinely putting in all the effort you can, on any given day, that's all that matters. Don't beat yourself up if you're not doing an hour a day in six weeks' time; this won't be for everyone. My Method is about finding what works personally for you – individual you – for ever. So hold yourself accountable and strive. But I want absolutely no guilt if you're falling short of perfection. Perfection is not necessary, and it's an illusion that serves no purpose.

So, for now, just focus on 15–20 minutes a day and let's see how you get on. You'll have days when you'll really struggle to put on your trainers, but once you get started and have some tunes blasting out, suddenly you'll want to do another round – this is more than often the case for me.

If you feel like you can or want to do more, simply repeat the 15-minute circuit again, with the same exercises; or pick another four exercises, to add variety. Remember: the more you put in, the more gratifying the transformation will be, in terms of speed, which is perhaps the greatest motivator of all. When you begin to feel and see the transformation, you'll want to do more – so dig deep and do the very best you can.

It's All about Pace

My workout method doesn't include time for faffing about and distraction. You're not to answer the phone, and you should keep all distractions to an absolute minimum. You don't have long, and I want you to focus on each and every movement.

There are days when I have a toddler hanging off my leg and I have to train to *Peppa Pig*. Just do what you need to do, but try to set a boundary with your family that this is *your* time and you are not to be disturbed.

By keeping the pace up, whilst you are toning your body for long-term results, you're burning fat at the most satisfying pace. By cardio-conditioning, you are killing two birds with one stone – and any distractions will negate the effects of this. So really do what you can to block out the noise around you.

You'll move swiftly between exercises, without taking breaks, as I want to keep your heart rate up – and the momentum of the workout. As you get more familiar with the moves, your pace and repetitions will increase within each one-minute slot.

Control Is Key

Whilst I want you to keep up the pace as you move through your workouts, each exercise should be completed with control and accuracy. Focus on your form and technique and you will get abundantly more from each move. In the first week, in particular, take your time to learn the precision of each movement, as it's the fine details that will make all the difference to your results and to preventing injury.

It is not a race against the clock, and you aren't going to be keeping count of how many repetitions you do each minute. Just work at a good pace and be sensible. Listen to your body and, if you are in any pain, stop.

Breathing

You have to breathe. During each exercise think about your breathing and concentrate on getting it into a good rhythm. It's all about rhythm. It's too easy to fall into the habit of holding on to your breath, so make sure that a good breathing technique is established as you begin. I prefer to breathe in on the easier part of the move and breathe out on the exertion – but do whatever works for you.

Controlling your breathing patterns as you train brings oxygen to your muscles when you need it and is crucial for focus – allowing your mind to really connect with your muscles. This sounds like hippy nonsense, but your muscles require your brain to engage with every move, to get the very best out of them.

Engage Your Core

You'll soon be aware that I've included specific exercises to challenge your core – the centre of your body and the area responsible for beautiful posture and healthy, functional movement – and this cannot be ignored.

I don't believe in doing thousands of crunches, in a bid for the perfect stomach. My total-body workouts are going to burn fat from all over your body, and it's actually working the body in unison and balance that will burn your abdominal fat, alongside the other pillars of my Method.

However, with every single exercise you do, I want you to **engage your core**. It should always be activated. Your brain will soon learn how to do this, without you even thinking about it; it just takes some practice and consistency.

To engage your core, simply pull in your pelvic-floor muscles (as if you are trying to stop the flow, mid-wee) and then gently pull in your belly button towards your spine. This will support your back and posture throughout each exercise, lessening the risk of injury and, most of all, speeding along your results.

Never, Ever Skip Your Warm-up

If you skip your warm-up, it's likely that you'll pick up a twinge at some point. It's essential that you spend five minutes mobilizing your muscles and joints and bringing your heart rate up gently, in preparation for your workout. If you're training early in the morning, remember that your body has been at rest for eight hours, so you may need to warm up for a little longer. If you've just power-walked home and are going straight into your workout, you'll already be partially warmed up, but you must still mobilize your joints for the workout ahead.

As with your main workout, simply complete each warm-up move for one minute and move between them nice and swiftly. Never force your range of motion – it will increase as the days go by; really listen to your body and don't try to force it beyond what you feel it is ready for. Only *you* can do this, and you will learn to connect with your body and know what it is capable of – it just takes a bit of time to tune in.

Never, ever skip your warm-up

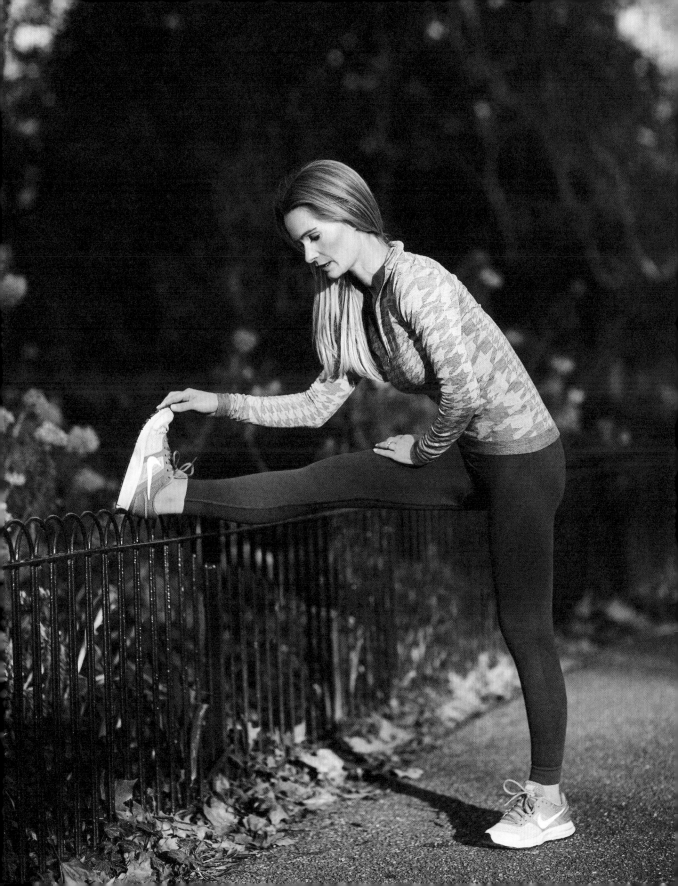

THE
EXERCISES

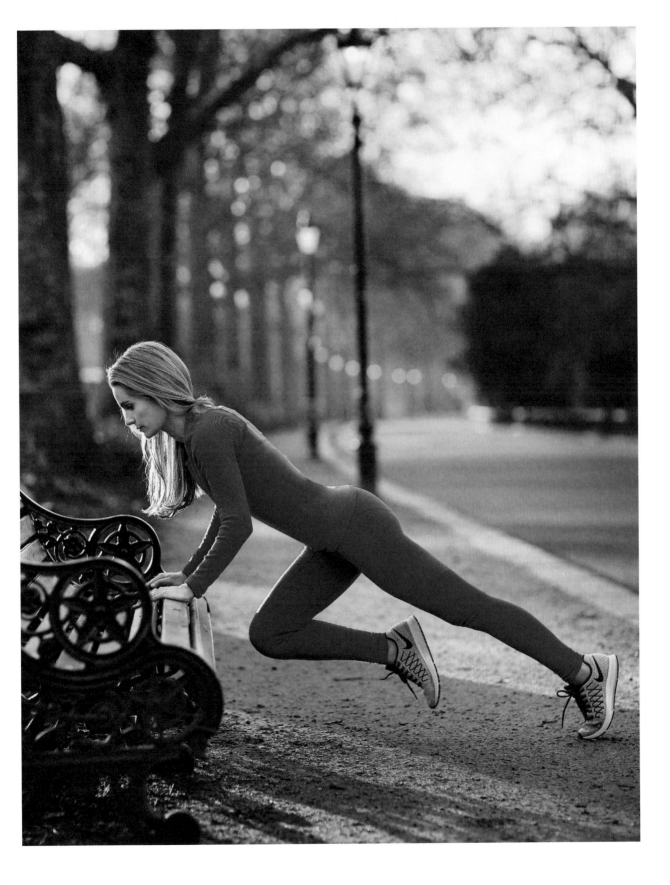

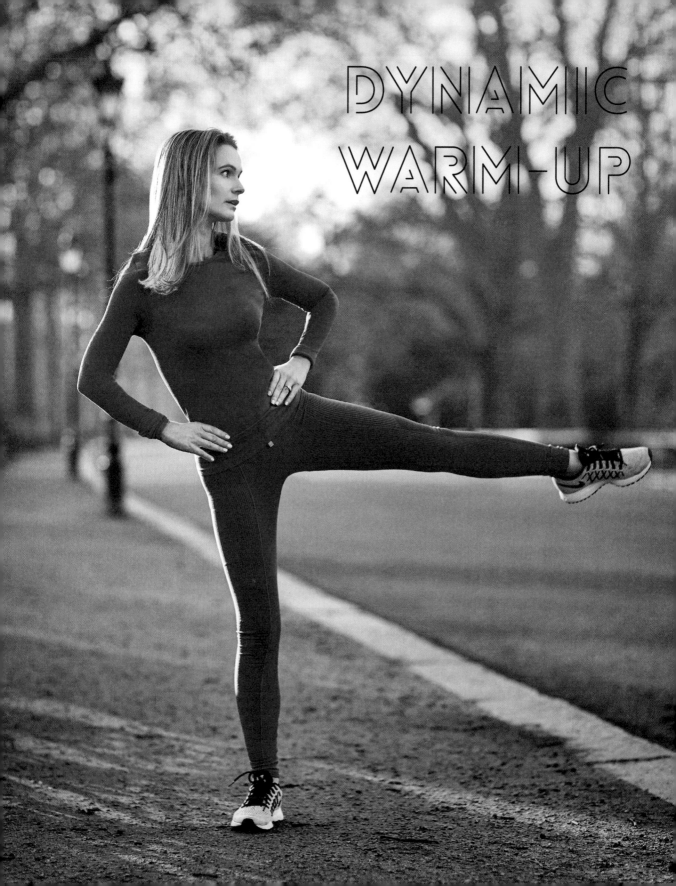

DYNAMIC WARM-UP

1. WARMING WINDMILLS

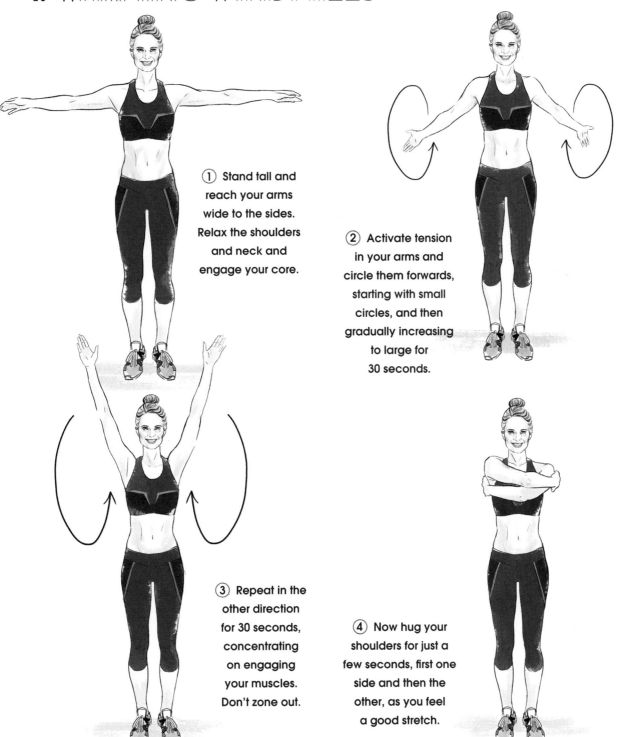

① Stand tall and reach your arms wide to the sides. Relax the shoulders and neck and engage your core.

② Activate tension in your arms and circle them forwards, starting with small circles, and then gradually increasing to large for 30 seconds.

③ Repeat in the other direction for 30 seconds, concentrating on engaging your muscles. Don't zone out.

④ Now hug your shoulders for just a few seconds, first one side and then the other, as you feel a good stretch.

2. SQUAT AND SHOULDER SLIDE

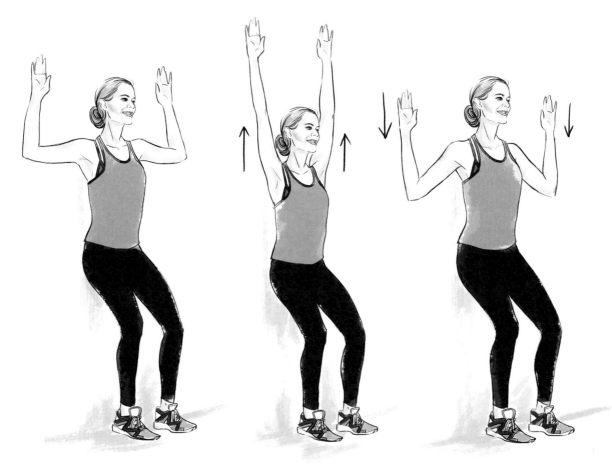

(1) Squat against a wall, at a height that you can hold for 1 minute, with your feet hip-width apart. Your knees must not extend beyond your toe line. Engage your core, ensuring your back, shoulders, arms and hands are in full contact with the wall. Your flexibility will dictate the height of your elbows in the starting position.

(2) Now slowly slide your arms upwards with concentration and control, maintaining contact with the wall, until your hands are fully extended above your head. Pull your belly button in towards the wall. Remember to focus on keeping your squat still and stable.

(3) With smooth control, lower your elbows back down to the starting position, keeping full contact with the wall, and keep repeating the motion with fluid and focused form. Keeping your belly button pulled into the wall whilst maintaining concentration is the secret here. Its harder than it looks!

3. WALKOUT WONDERS

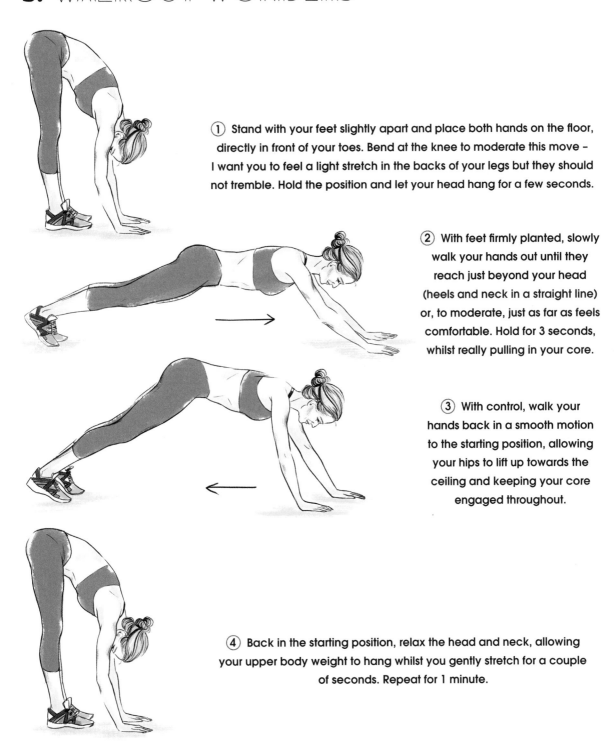

1. Stand with your feet slightly apart and place both hands on the floor, directly in front of your toes. Bend at the knee to moderate this move – I want you to feel a light stretch in the backs of your legs but they should not tremble. Hold the position and let your head hang for a few seconds.

2. With feet firmly planted, slowly walk your hands out until they reach just beyond your head (heels and neck in a straight line) or, to moderate, just as far as feels comfortable. Hold for 3 seconds, whilst really pulling in your core.

3. With control, walk your hands back in a smooth motion to the starting position, allowing your hips to lift up towards the ceiling and keeping your core engaged throughout.

4. Back in the starting position, relax the head and neck, allowing your upper body weight to hang whilst you gently stretch for a couple of seconds. Repeat for 1 minute.

4. LATERALLY LEAN

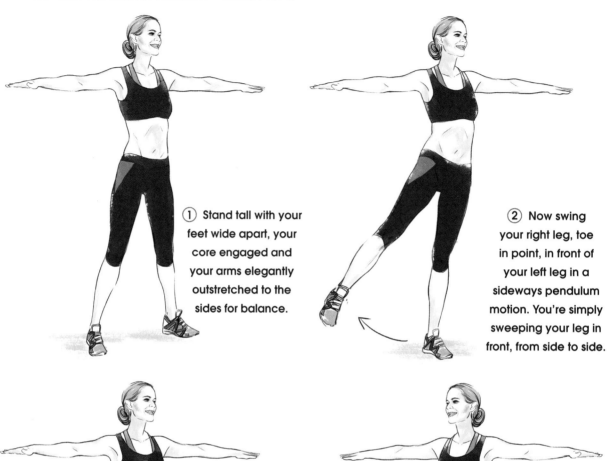

① Stand tall with your feet wide apart, your core engaged and your arms elegantly outstretched to the sides for balance.

② Now swing your right leg, toe in point, in front of your left leg in a sideways pendulum motion. You're simply sweeping your leg in front, from side to side.

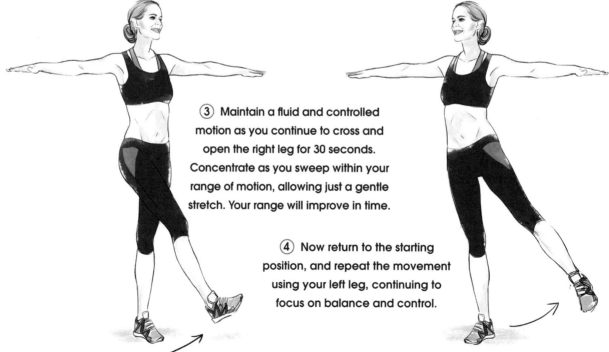

③ Maintain a fluid and controlled motion as you continue to cross and open the right leg for 30 seconds. Concentrate as you sweep within your range of motion, allowing just a gentle stretch. Your range will improve in time.

④ Now return to the starting position, and repeat the movement using your left leg, continuing to focus on balance and control.

5. MOBILIZING MARCH

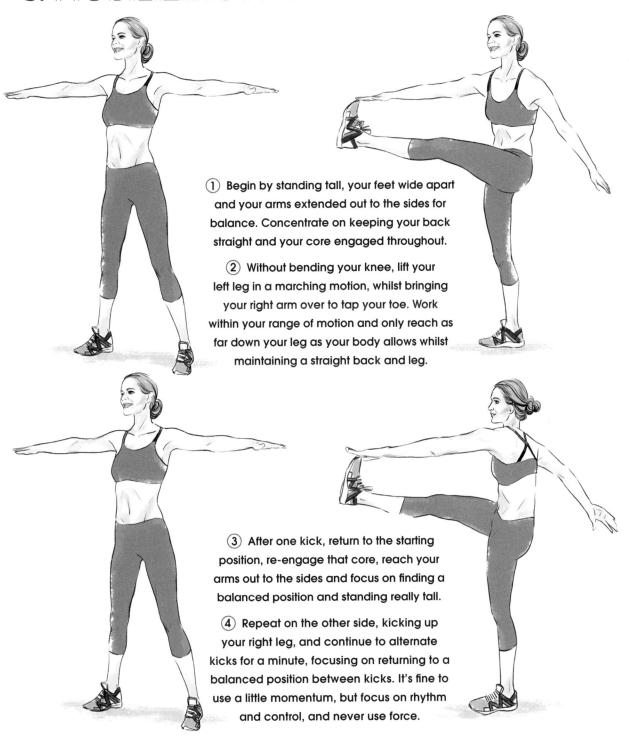

① Begin by standing tall, your feet wide apart and your arms extended out to the sides for balance. Concentrate on keeping your back straight and your core engaged throughout.

② Without bending your knee, lift your left leg in a marching motion, whilst bringing your right arm over to tap your toe. Work within your range of motion and only reach as far down your leg as your body allows whilst maintaining a straight back and leg.

③ After one kick, return to the starting position, re-engage that core, reach your arms out to the sides and focus on finding a balanced position and standing really tall.

④ Repeat on the other side, kicking up your right leg, and continue to alternate kicks for a minute, focusing on returning to a balanced position between kicks. It's fine to use a little momentum, but focus on rhythm and control, and never use force.

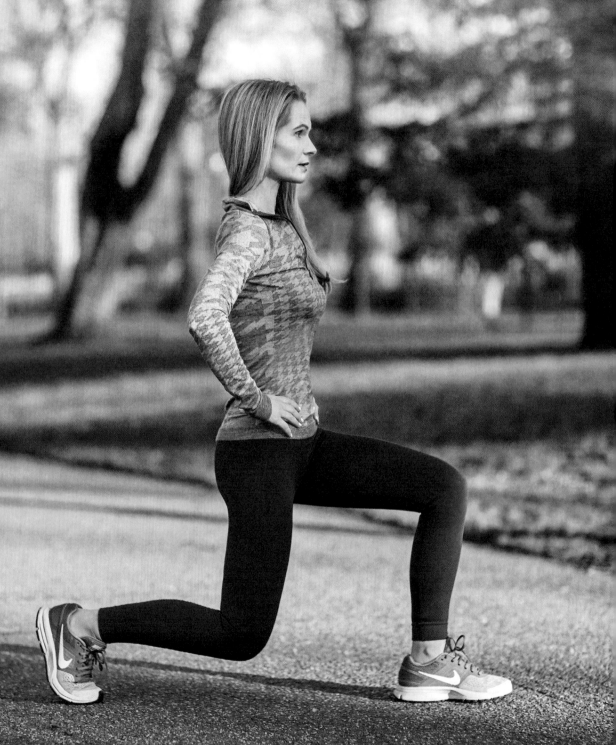

1. SLINKY SIDEYS

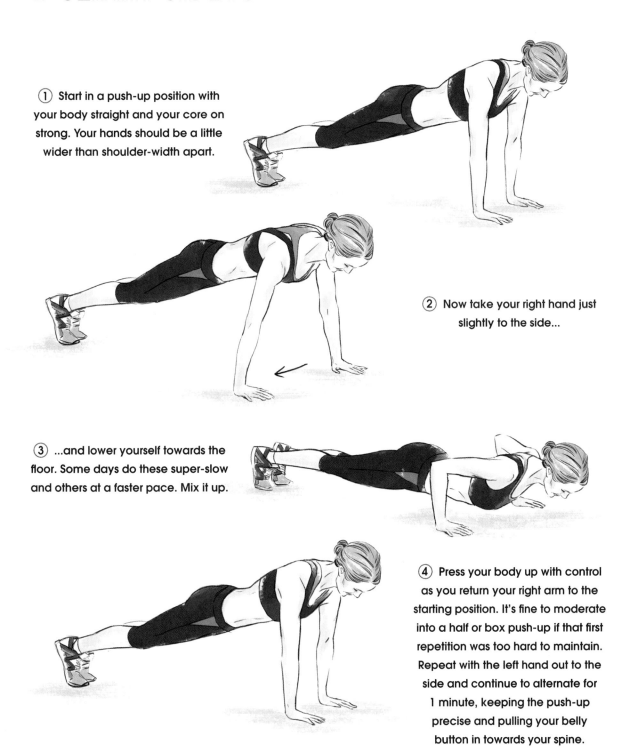

① Start in a push-up position with your body straight and your core on strong. Your hands should be a little wider than shoulder-width apart.

② Now take your right hand just slightly to the side...

③ ...and lower yourself towards the floor. Some days do these super-slow and others at a faster pace. Mix it up.

④ Press your body up with control as you return your right arm to the starting position. It's fine to moderate into a half or box push-up if that first repetition was too hard to maintain. Repeat with the left hand out to the side and continue to alternate for 1 minute, keeping the push-up precise and pulling your belly button in towards your spine.

2. SIDE-PLANK ROTATION

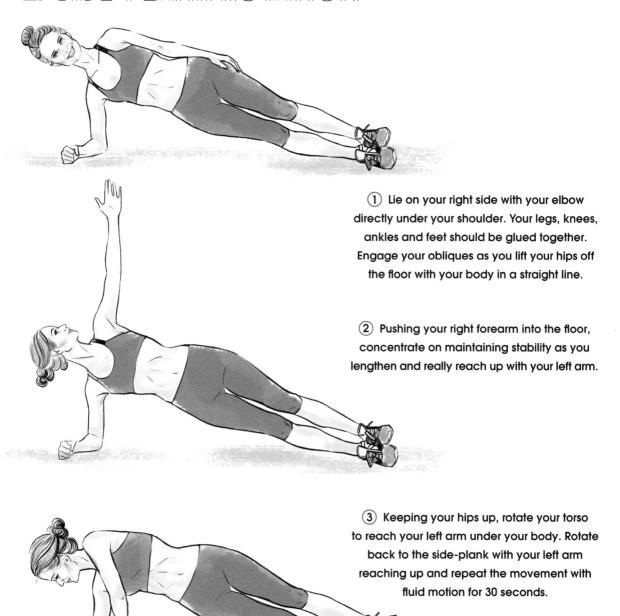

① Lie on your right side with your elbow directly under your shoulder. Your legs, knees, ankles and feet should be glued together. Engage your obliques as you lift your hips off the floor with your body in a straight line.

② Pushing your right forearm into the floor, concentrate on maintaining stability as you lengthen and really reach up with your left arm.

③ Keeping your hips up, rotate your torso to reach your left arm under your body. Rotate back to the side-plank with your left arm reaching up and repeat the movement with fluid motion for 30 seconds.

④ Now lie on your left side and repeat the move for another 30 seconds.

3. SQUATS ON FIRE

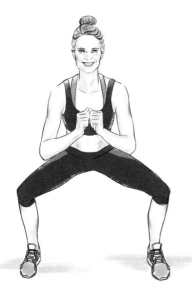

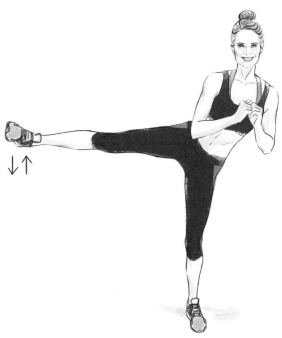

① Stand with your feet wide apart and sit back into a squat with thighs parallel to the ground. Ensure your knees do not cross over your toe line. Your hands should be clenched at the centre of your body.

② As you stand up, really push up through the left heel and extend your right leg into a side-kick, pulsing up and down at the top for 5 slow repetitions.

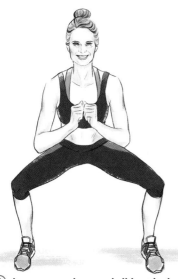

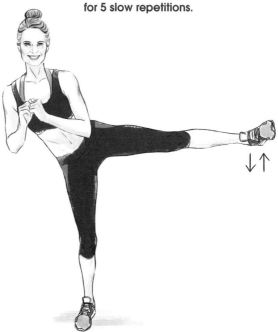

③ Lower your leg and sit back down into the squat, preparing to push up again through the opposite heel.

④ Repeat with the left leg and continue alternating until you have completed a full minute.

4. PUNCHY SUMO SQUAT

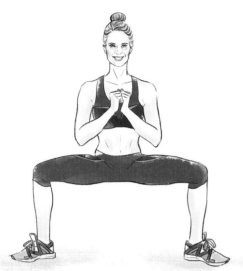

① Sit in a wide squat with your toes turned out at a 45-degree angle and your hands clenched at the centre of your body. Your back should be straight and your core engaged.

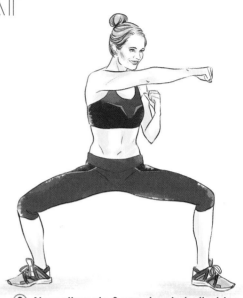

② Now alternate 8 punches to both sides. Concentrate on adding tension to your punches and maintaining the stability of your squat.

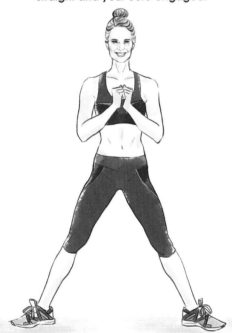

③ Push up to a standing position and return your fists to the centre, ensuring that your belly button is pulled in and your back straight.

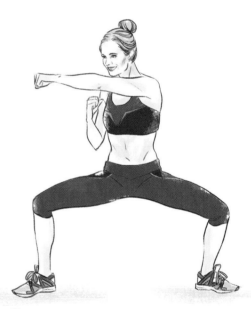

④ Sit back down into the squat and perform another 8 alternating punches, then stand tall, squat down and repeat until you complete 1 minute.

5. THE PERFECT PLANK

① Start with your knees on the floor, hip-width apart, and lower down on to your forearms, which should be shoulder-width apart with fingers pointing forwards in line with your elbows.

② Now step your feet back so that your body forms a straight line from your head to your heels. Draw your belly button in towards your spine but avoid tensing your neck and shoulders.

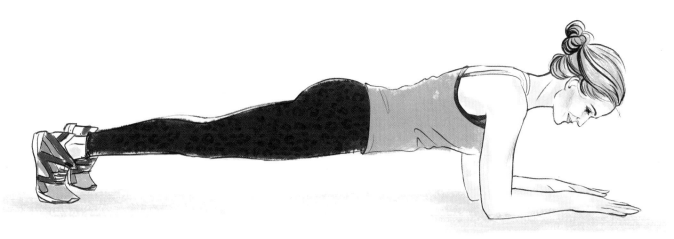

③ Concentrate on drawing your shoulder blades down your back and increase the distance between your shoulders and ears. Don't allow your back to droop. Keep your hips in line with your shoulders.

④ Hold the position for a minute if possible, but take a break if you need to – you'll soon be able to hold this pose for longer than a minute.

6. GLOBAL PLANK

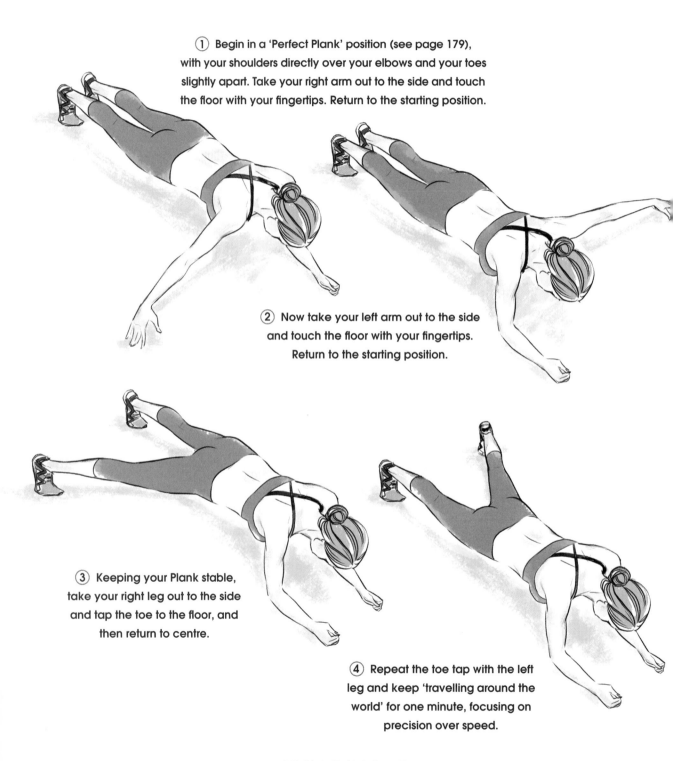

① Begin in a 'Perfect Plank' position (see page 179), with your shoulders directly over your elbows and your toes slightly apart. Take your right arm out to the side and touch the floor with your fingertips. Return to the starting position.

② Now take your left arm out to the side and touch the floor with your fingertips. Return to the starting position.

③ Keeping your Plank stable, take your right leg out to the side and tap the toe to the floor, and then return to centre.

④ Repeat the toe tap with the left leg and keep 'travelling around the world' for one minute, focusing on precision over speed.

7. WALKING LUNGE WITH OVERHEAD REACH

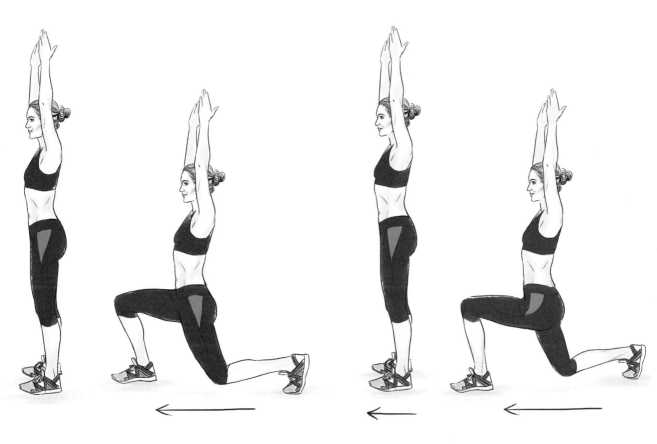

① Stand beautifully tall with your core engaged and extend both arms above your head, shoulders relaxed and the palms of your hands facing one another. Hold your chest high and gently squeeze your shoulder blades together throughout.

② Take a step forwards with your right leg whilst lifting up onto the ball of the back foot. Bend your knees and drop your hips down towards the floor, keeping the back knee off the floor and making sure that the front knee doesn't extend beyond the toe line.

③ Now push up with your front leg and walk your back foot forwards, returning to the starting position. Focus on standing tall, relaxing your shoulders and keeping your neck in line with your spine.

④ Now lunge forward with the left leg, and then return to the starting position. Continue alternating legs and walking forwards for 1 minute, focusing on form rather than speed.

8. PIKE PUSH-UP

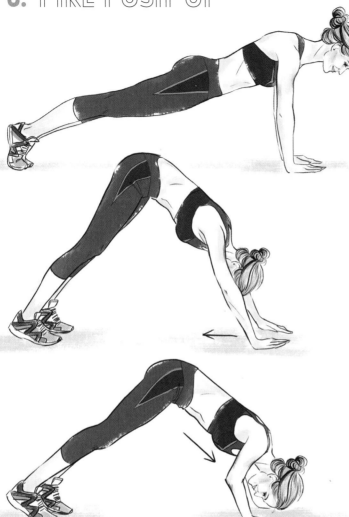

① Begin in a classic push-up position, with your hands shoulder-width apart and your fingers pointing slightly inwards.

② Keeping your legs straight, walk your hands back, so that your hips are reaching to the ceiling and your body is in an upside-down V-shape. Ensure that your arms are in line with your spine and are reaching straight out from your shoulders.

③ As you push your hips up, with your heels slightly raised, bend your elbows to the sides and slowly lower your head towards the floor into a small push-up.

④ Now press back up. Maintain this form and repeat the push-ups for 1 minute, taking a break if you need to.

9. CLASSIC JUMP SQUAT

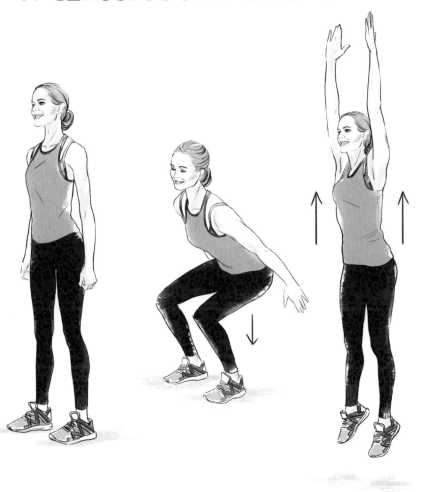
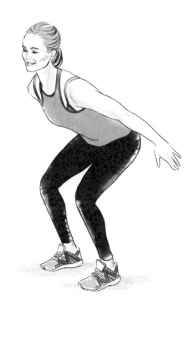

① Stand with your feet hip-width apart, your toes forwards and your core engaged. Focus your mind – this plyometric movement requires concentration and beautiful control.

② Begin by squatting down to a seated position, with your arms by your sides and your core engaged, and prepare to jump.

③ Now jump up with a real push off the floor and reach your arms overhead, keeping your body in a straight line and your core engaged.

④ Land as softly as you can and with careful control. Next sit back into the squat, before repeating the plyometric jump. Focus on form and rhythm until you've really mastered the move, and only then increase the number of repetitions that you do in 1 minute.

10. SLIM SIDE-LUNGE

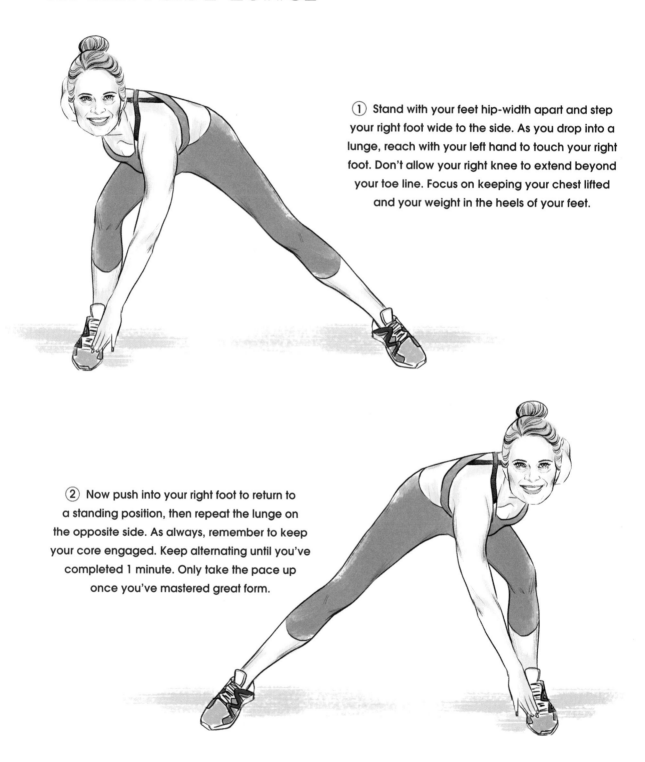

① Stand with your feet hip-width apart and step your right foot wide to the side. As you drop into a lunge, reach with your left hand to touch your right foot. Don't allow your right knee to extend beyond your toe line. Focus on keeping your chest lifted and your weight in the heels of your feet.

② Now push into your right foot to return to a standing position, then repeat the lunge on the opposite side. As always, remember to keep your core engaged. Keep alternating until you've completed 1 minute. Only take the pace up once you've mastered great form.

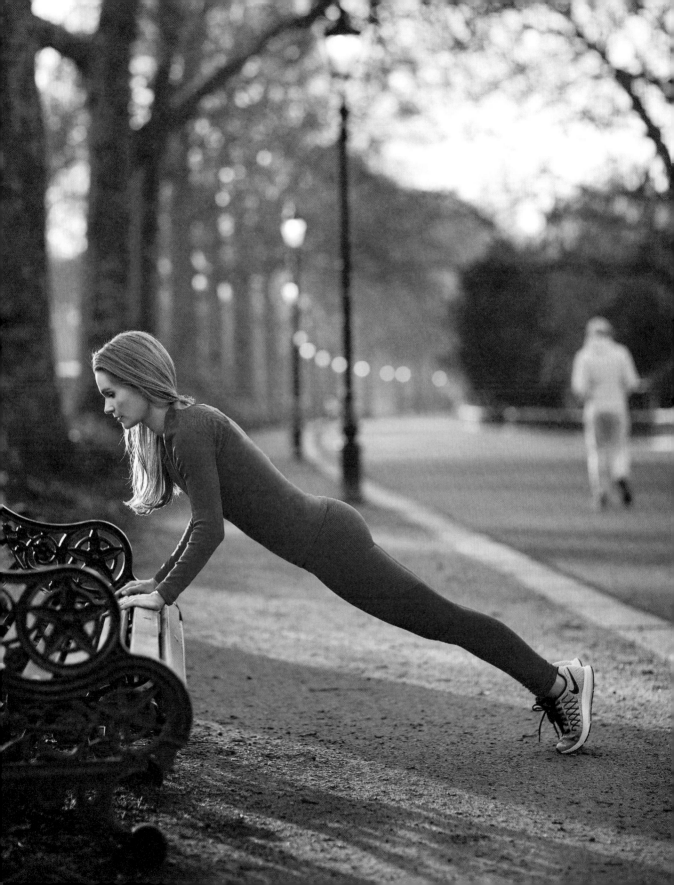

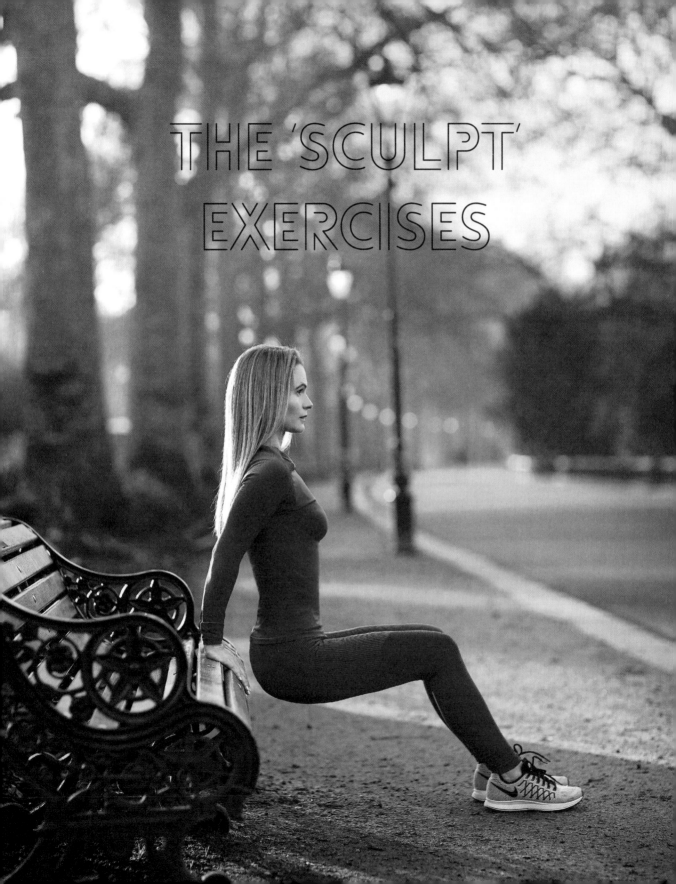

THE 'SCULPT' EXERCISES

1. CLAMS ON FIRE

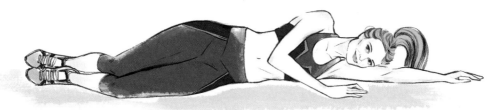

① Lying on your left side with your left arm extended beneath your head in line with your spine, rest your right hand on the floor in front of you. Keep your spine straight and aligned with the fronts of your hips, bringing your knees forwards and keeping your hips stacked as if your back were against a wall.

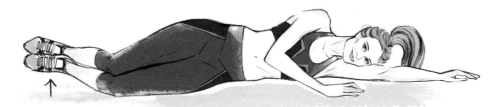

② Keeping your knees and toes glued together, lift your feet up off the floor. Your shoulders and hips should remain neatly stacked and your spine elongated throughout.

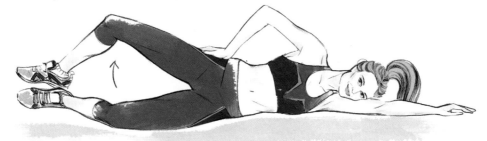

③ Now raise the top right knee, so that your legs open like a clam. Place your right hand on your glutes and feel the muscle really contract as you pulse in this position for 30 seconds.

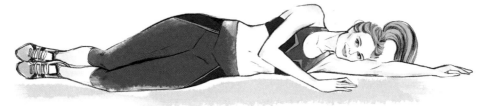

④ Release the top knee back down and then lower your feet to the floor. Turn over to work the other side. Remember to keep your hips and shoulders stacked and your spine elongated, and avoid leaning back. Focus on the buttocks and ensure they are doing all the lifting.

2. TONE AND TWIST

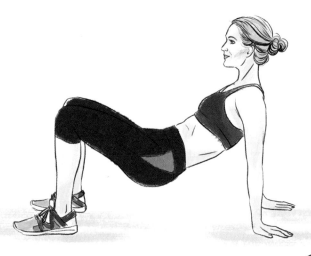

(1) Sit on the floor with your knees bent, feet firmly planted, hands below your shoulders, and fingers pointing behind you. Lift your bottom up off the floor a few inches. This is your starting position.

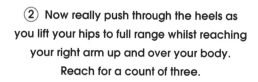

(2) Now really push through the heels as you lift your hips to full range whilst reaching your right arm up and over your body. Reach for a count of three.

(3) Slowly release and return to the starting position.

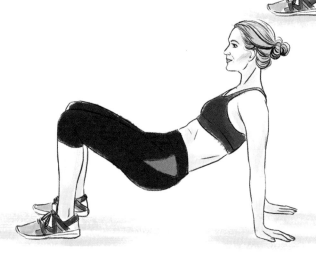

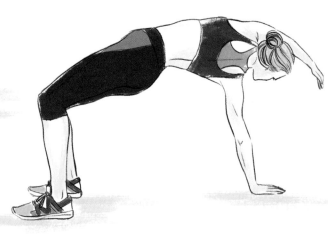

(4) Now reach the left arm across and over your body, holding for a count of three. Keep alternating sides for 1 minute, focusing on fluidity and control.

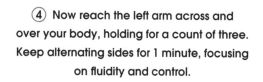

3. B AND B BURNERS

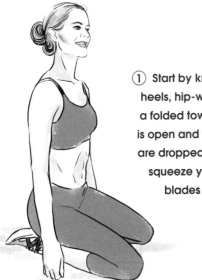

① Start by kneeling on your heels, hip-width apart, on a folded towel. Your chest is open and your shoulders are dropped as you gently squeeze your shoulder blades together.

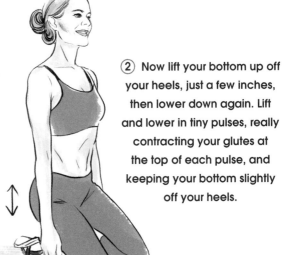

② Now lift your bottom up off your heels, just a few inches, then lower down again. Lift and lower in tiny pulses, really contracting your glutes at the top of each pulse, and keeping your bottom slightly off your heels.

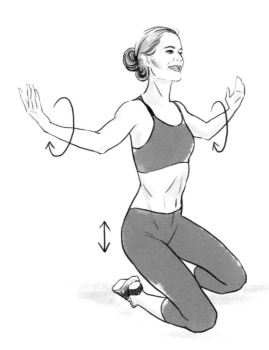

③ Keeping your lower pulses going, take your arms out to the sides with palms facing up and elbows soft. Engage the biceps as you begin to circle your arms within a small range, alternating circling backwards and forwards for a count of 10. Focus on coordinating your arm circles and glute pulses with control for 1 minute.

4. TEENY TRICEPS

① Sit on the floor with your knees bent and your hands positioned directly below your shoulders, with your fingers pointing forwards.

② Lift your bottom off the floor, just a few inches, and extend your right leg at a 45-degree angle from the floor.

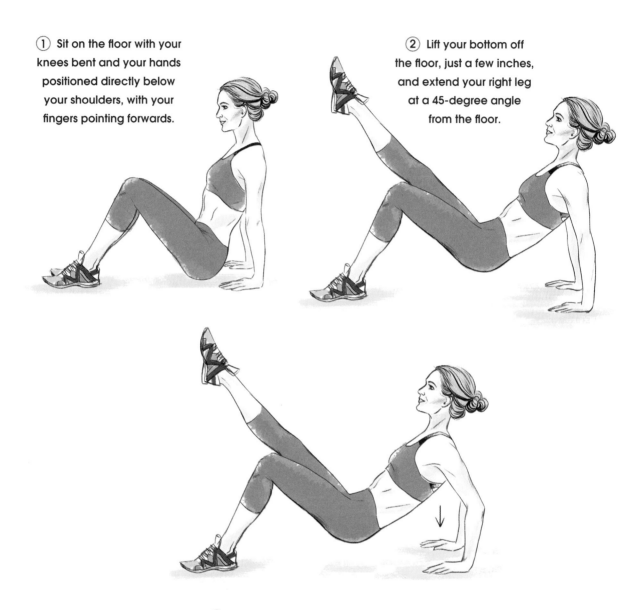

③ With your bottom and core really activated, perform little triceps dips, with your elbows neatly tucked in. Repeat for 30 seconds.

④ Now swap sides and complete a further 30 seconds of triceps dips with your left leg extended.

5. GRACEFUL GLUTES

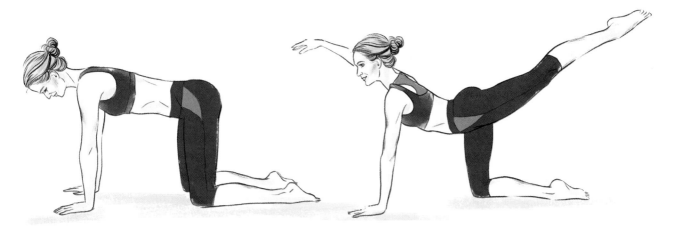

① Start by kneeling on your hands and knees, with your neck relaxed and in line with your spine. It's essential that you really pull your belly button into the spine throughout this movement, to protect your lower back.

② Now straighten and lengthen your left leg and lift it upwards in point as you focus on your buttocks doing the lift. Simultaneously lift your right arm and keep it long and graceful. Hold the position for a count of three.

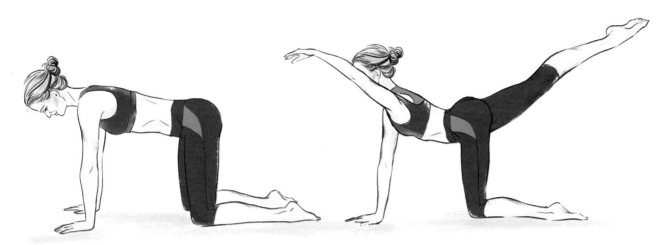

③ Release and return to the starting position, relaxing your neck back into neutral and re-engaging the core.

④ Repeat on the other side and then continue to alternate the movement for 1 minute, keeping it fluid and graceful. Listen to your body and don't force it beyond your natural range of motion.

6. DOWNWARD DOG, UPWARD BUM

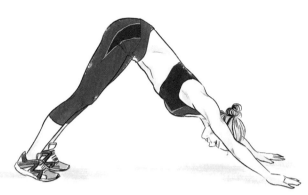

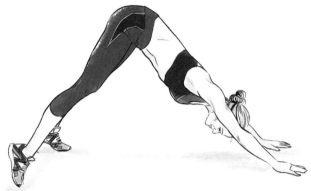

① Begin in a Downward Dog pose with your body in an A shape. Your arms should be straight, fingers pointing forwards and weight spread evenly through your hands. Relax your upper back and head. Gently straighten your legs without locking.

② Press the floor away from you using your straight arms as you lift through your pelvis and shift your weight to your left leg and extend your right leg to the right, with foot pointed. Keep lengthening your spine.

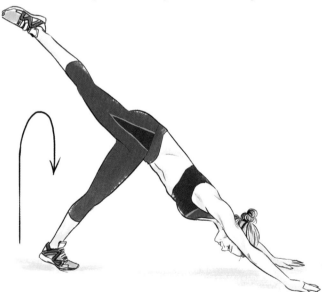

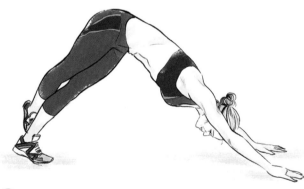

③ Lift the right leg up from the buttocks and create a straight line between your hands and your right foot. Keep your arms and legs firm, chest broad and core engaged throughout.

④ Sweep your right leg over your left in a semicircle then lower your right toe to the side of your left foot. Continue the movement, alternating legs, for 1 minute. To release, exhale as you gently bend your knees and come back to your hands and knees.

7. HIGH AND LOW TOE TAPS

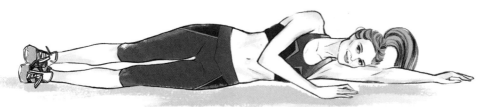

① Positioning a chair at your feet, lie down on the left side of your body, spine extended, with hips stacked and legs glued together. Your right hand should be placed gently in front of your torso.

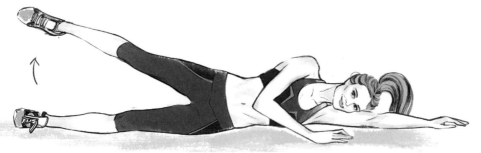

② Lift your right leg, toe in point, to the height of the chair seat. Keeping your toe in point, lift the leg higher and in a graceful circle.

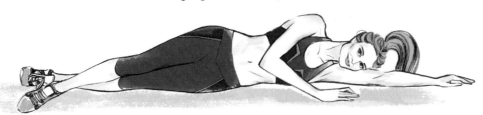

③ Lower your right leg, toe still in point, to toe-tap the floor a few inches to one side of the chair.

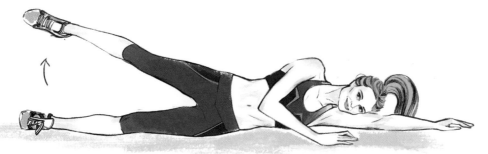

④ Focusing on keeping your torso stable and your body relaxed, draw the right leg back up in a circular motion to the height of the chair. Repeat this movement, without stopping, for 30 seconds, then roll over and repeat on the other side. Focus on your core stabilizing you, so that you can relax the supporting arm and maintain a relaxed upper body.

8. PULSING PRETZEL

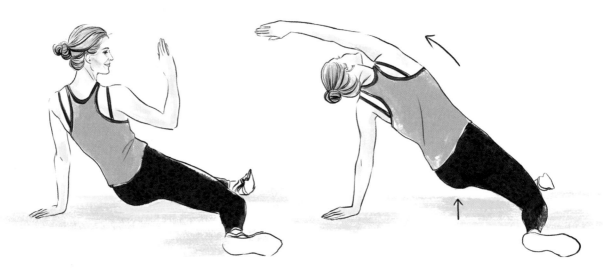

① Arrange yourself on the floor with both of your knees bent at 90 degrees, your left leg in front of you and your right leg behind you. Now lean forwards a little and place your left hand on the floor next to your left hip.

② Keep your knees on the floor and use your buttocks and obliques to scoop your torso up off the floor as your right arm reaches up and over your body.

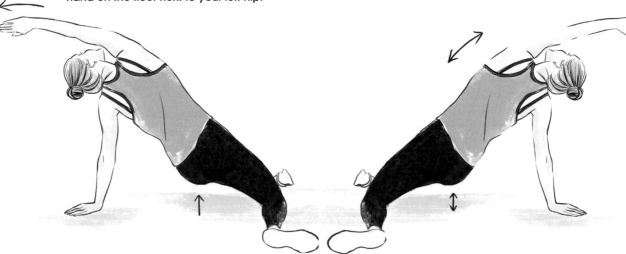

③ Now pulse for 30 seconds at the top of the movement, with beautiful control. Keep the range of motion small and precise.

④ Release down, swap to the other side and repeat the exercise until you've completed your full minute.

9. PASSÉ POINTS

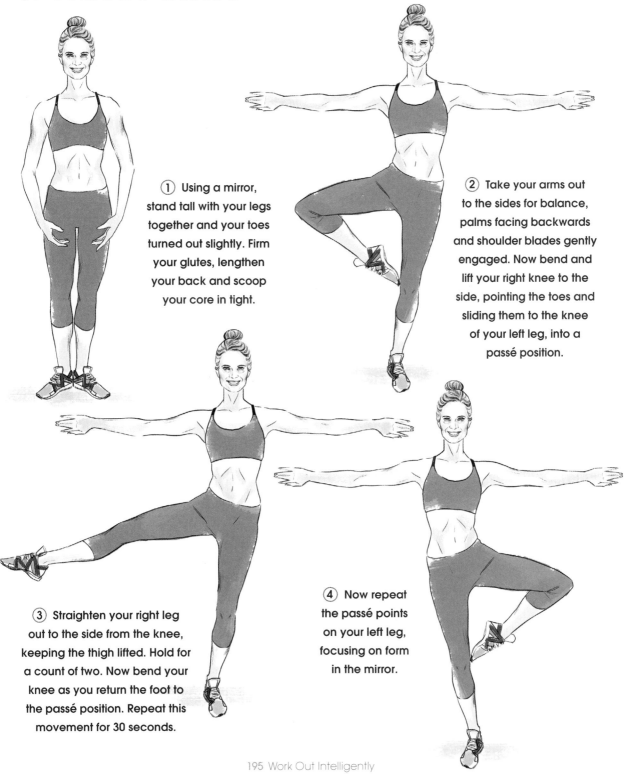

① Using a mirror, stand tall with your legs together and your toes turned out slightly. Firm your glutes, lengthen your back and scoop your core in tight.

② Take your arms out to the sides for balance, palms facing backwards and shoulder blades gently engaged. Now bend and lift your right knee to the side, pointing the toes and sliding them to the knee of your left leg, into a passé position.

③ Straighten your right leg out to the side from the knee, keeping the thigh lifted. Hold for a count of two. Now bend your knee as you return the foot to the passé position. Repeat this movement for 30 seconds.

④ Now repeat the passé points on your left leg, focusing on form in the mirror.

10. TRI AND AB POINTS

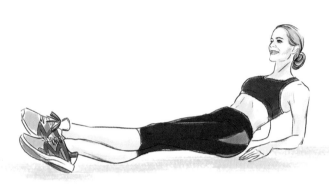

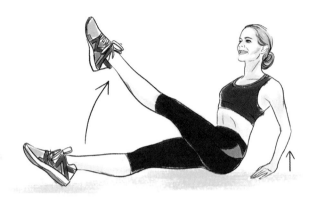

① Begin by leaning back onto your elbows with your forearms and hands glued to the floor and both legs extended straight in front of you. Your chest should be wide open, your shoulders positioned above your elbows and your core engaged. Now lift your left leg and cross it over your right.

② Push into your hands, straightening your arms and lifting your chest as you simultaneously lift your left leg towards your chest. Draw your belly button in towards your back and hold this position for a count of three.

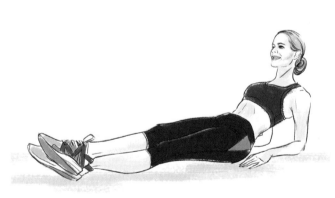

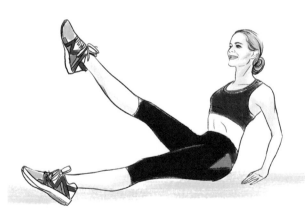

③ Using your triceps and core, release slowly back to the starting position. Now lift your right leg and cross it over your left.

④ Repeat the move on the opposite side, and then continue alternating for 1 minute. Keep drawing your belly button in towards your back and visualize your triceps lifting and lowering you.

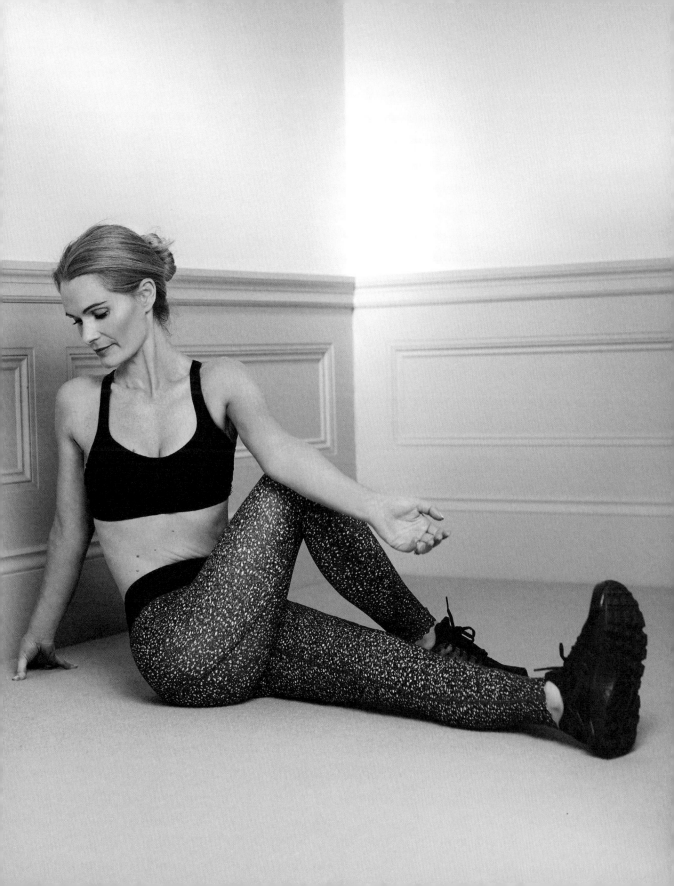

THE PROGRAMME

I've taken you through the building blocks of my Method in detail, and now it's time to put it all into action. I've explained the science and crammed every bit of it into one simple programme. You'll notice that this section is short – and that's a good thing. Simplicity is brilliance and we don't need to overcomplicate things: this is about do-ability and longevity.

You are going to take the most direct route to the body you choose for yourself. The direct route is the easiest route and you're going to **start once and just not stop**, until you get a result that truly takes your breath away.

The Transform Phase is going to infuse you with motivation, enthusiasm and determination to succeed, as the pace of results consistently propels you forward. When you see your body morphing before your eyes, you're going to want to keep going and stay on track. Your motivation will morph into habits greater than any temptation in your path. And besides, the Transform Phase you do **ONCE** and it's a temporary situation – the cupcakes and Chablis will still be there at the end of your transformation. They're not going anywhere, but you most certainly are.

In this phase, you are going to shed body fat at the most impressive rate whilst sculpting a beautifully toned body. When the two come together at the end of your transformation, you'll be in the best shape of your life.

Your body will go into a fat-burning zone where muscle is preserved and all the weight that you lose is pure fat.

I've thought of everything to make sure that you hang on to every ounce of muscle mass you have, and then add some more – because it's your muscle tone that will *keep* you lean and sculpt your body slim.

During your Transform Phase you're going to put in extra effort. I want you to make your programme an absolute priority. You'll only need to do this phase once, before you maintain your results for ever in the Lifestyle Plan. It may be that you need to do two or three rounds, but – given what the prize is and that it needs just one big push – isn't it worth giving it your absolute all? Once you've got the body and the habit, it will be a breeze.

Really get behind Transform, take pride in every meal and throw all you can possibly muster into every single workout. Put your heart, soul and backside into it. Do it all, get your sleep, look after yourself better than you ever have before and give yourself the focus and attention that you deserve. You are the priority now. Don't let work or family commitments or problems hold you back – you'll be a happier, stronger, fitter and more patient person once your transformation is complete. It's not selfish to put yourself first – it's crucial. Remember you are now top priority.

Nothing worth having comes without effort, but my Method is as stress-free, simple and swift as it gets. So it's as time-effective as it possibly can be – but you *are* still going to have to work for it.

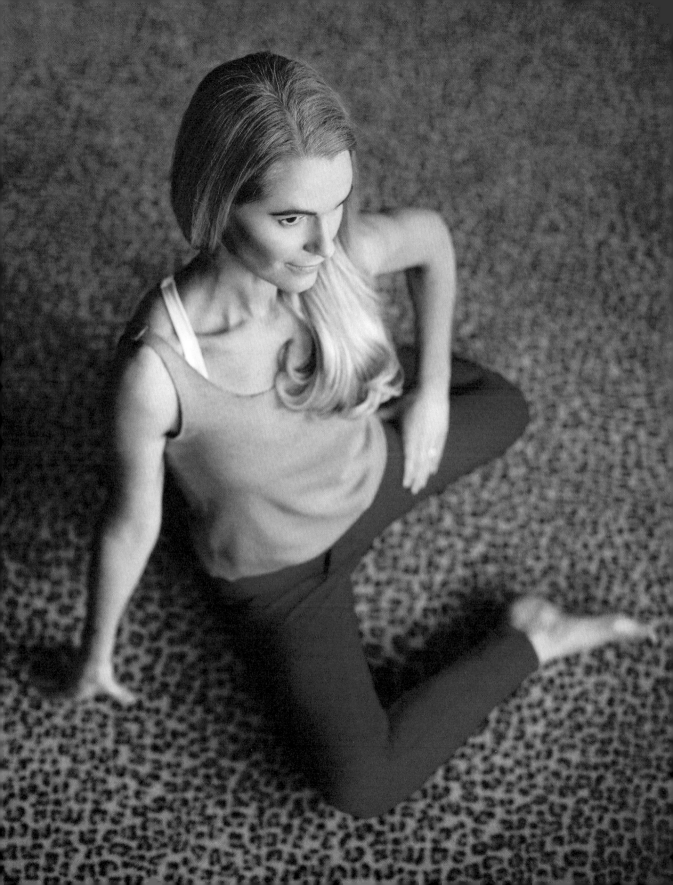

Transform

In the Introduction I talked about my programme being like a new dance that you are going to learn. In the Transform Phase you are going to practise the steps that will give you beautiful results, and the habits that will help you to sustain it for ever.

To get the best possible results, you're going to master these steps in a small area. We call this the 'inner circle'. When you're in this inner circle you're going to be burning fat, building muscle tone and creating your New Normal.

Once you reach your goal, I'll show you how to relax into the celebrations of life without a moment's guilt, as you dance between the circles in perfect balance. But for now we're going to focus on this fabulously effective, fat-burning inner circle.

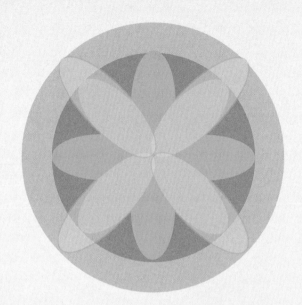

HERE'S HOW YOU'RE GOING TO STAY IN THE INNER CIRCLE:

MINDSET

★ Adopt a positive mindset and assume success

★ Make time for simple pleasures every single day

★ Deal with and dissolve all your worries

★ Keep positive, inspiring company

1

LIFESTYLE

★ Declutter your surroundings

★ Digital detox after 9pm every night

★ Sleep 7 hours a night

★ Take a 'brain-nap' for 20 minutes a day

2

NUTRITION

★ Eat 3 meals and 2 snacks per day. You have a choice of 80 recipes, each super simple and quick to prepare

★ Start your day with 'Lemonize' and stay well hydrated throughout

3

EXERCISE

★ Weave activity into your everyday, with an absolute minimum of 10,000 steps per day. Aim as high as you can

★ Complete a minimum of 15 minutes of my Louise Parker Method home workouts

4

On each day of the programme I want you to use the simple visualization of the inner circle to help focus you on achieving your ultimate goal. Treasure each daily success and take pride as the days of learning this new dance in the inner circle add up. Ink them, think them – whatever works for you.

Visualize 42 circles in total (your six-week programme of seven days) and enjoy the satisfaction of ticking off each day, each tick transporting you further towards your goal and setting your habits.

Because the programme is incredibly practical, time-efficient and supports your willpower, once you've decided to start, it really is easier to stay in the circle than you might think. Simply focus on getting your head on the pillow at the end of each day, having stayed in the inner circle.

Don't overthink it – take it one meal at a time and one workout at a time. Don't worry about how long it's going to take you to reach your goal. The time is going to pass anyway; just know that you're taking the most direct route.

After spending 42 days in your inner circle, you'll have the most amazing transformation: beautiful results and new habits that will last a lifetime.

It's simple, intelligent and beautifully effective.

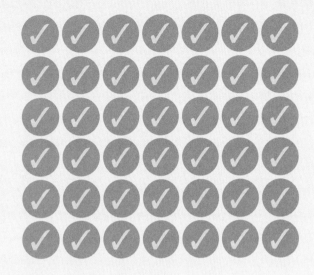

Don't Pick-and-Mix

Each aspect of the programme is there for a reason and has been adapted and refined to help you to achieve the best results possible. So please don't 'pick-and-mix' the aspects that you do – you need to do them all, as the programme's success is down to the sum of its parts. When you put it all together over a number of weeks, the results will amaze you.

In this phase, you are going to shed body fat at the most impressive rate, whilst sculpting a beautifully toned body. When the two come together at the end of your transformation, you'll be in the best shape of your life

Before Your Programme

Mental and practical preparation is crucial to your success. You are going to start strong, prepared and assuming success. Start once and do not stop until you've reached your goal.

Prepare

★ **Place your order** and set your goals (see right).

★ **Be accountable** to yourself and a group of supportive friends (see right). You are stronger together.

★ **Blitz your cupboards, fridge and freezer** – take your junk food to a food bank; you won't be needing it, and your kids can go without until your new lifestyle becomes a habit; it'll do them good too.

★ **Make a list of store-cupboard ingredients** that you'll need and take pride in arranging your goodies – use jars you love and keep the fridge beautifully arranged.

★ **Plan when to do your food shops** – in person or online at least twice a week – and place it in your diary.

★ **Ensure you've a couple of ready-prepared meals** in the fridge or freezer, so that you are never caught out.

★ **Spend 10 minutes mentally planning the next days' meals** – there's no need to put aside a whole day preparing them, but do get into the habit of mindfulness and daily organization.

★ **Put your daily workouts in your diary** and don't move them. Choose a time when you are less likely to have to abort, such as first thing in the morning or as soon as you get home from work. Think habit.

★ **Make sure you've got three workout outfits** that make you feel fabulous. If not, invest in workout wear that puts a spring in your step and that you'd be happy to be seen in by your ex-boyfriend. How you feel matters.

★ **Take your measurements and some 'Before' pictures**. You'll regret not doing this at the end of the programme, if you don't; so as scary as it may feel, just do it.

To use a cliché: if you fail to plan, you plan to fail. Don't wake up one morning and stumble into the programme with a false start and nothing in the fridge. Hot bodies don't happen by accident, and they do take some planning. Remember that the effort lessens, once you're at your goal and the programme has just become your lifestyle. I barely have to think about it at all any more – certainly no more so than anyone who has to cook food in order to survive.

Place Your Order

★ **Decide what you want to achieve**, in a specific and tangible way.

★ **Dream big and make a list** of at least five goals; ink them.

It's so important that you set clear, specific and tangible goals. Write down at least five bullet points describing what you would like to gain from the Method – and make sure that you dig deeper than simply 'weight loss'. Now tear it up and have another go, this time being 30 per cent more ambitious. Almost everyone we coach exceeds their expectations and sets their goals far too low, saying, 'I just wanted to be realistic'. In our world, phenomenal results are a reality, so aiming low is just doing yourself a disservice.

Be Accountable

You'll dramatically improve your results by making yourself accountable to someone other than yourself. Ultimately, what matters is that you are pleased with your progress, but checking in and helping someone other than yourself will also help you stick to the path. **Give help away and it will come back to you tenfold.**

Tribal Transformation

If you've a handful of friends or family that you know would love to transform once and for all, get them to join you. Gather up between four and eight of you and set up a weekly time to meet to encourage each other along and share your results of the week. Make sure that you set a regular time when you can all relax and be undistracted. You can be based anywhere in the world, but still help each other along. You're likely to have the odd challenge and the occasional week when it feels harder than other times, but there will always be a few of you feeling really optimistic – and this can only encourage you. Resolve not to moan, and to put a positive spin on things – a few ground rules can really help to keep your meetings constructive. Remember: it's about ending dieting and changing your mindset, and not just about transforming your body.

Sharing results, tips and encouragement really helps, and you are far more likely to exceed your goals if you support each other. This support is such an important factor in the success of the Louise Parker programmes, so don't overlook this as something that doesn't apply to you.

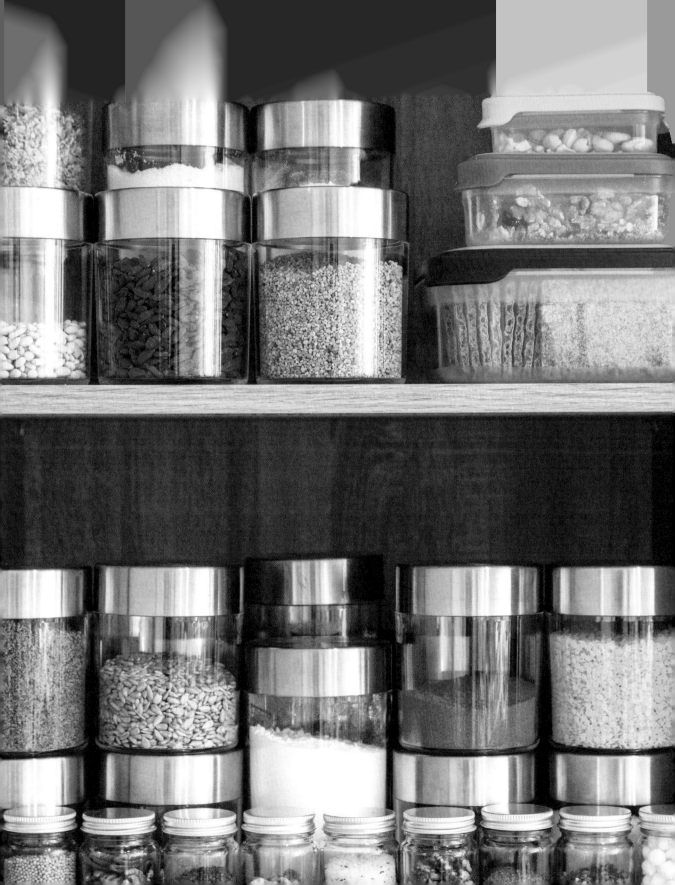

How to Measure your Transformation

'Before' & 'After' Photographs

Photographs are simply the best way of measuring your progress and I highly recommend taking some before you start, and every three weeks into each cycle of Transform (you need to give your body a little time to adjust, enough for your critical eye to be proud of). Either ask someone to do this for you, or take a selfie in front of a long mirror. Get your whole body in and take three pictures: one full-frontal, one to the side and then turn around and take a picture of the back of you in the mirror, using the selfie button on your phone. (If you're not up to speed with these gadgets, then you'll have to dig deep and ask your nearest and dearest to help you.) Make sure you wear a swimsuit, bikini or, at the very least, tight leggings (not black) and a really fitted top or sports bra. You need to be able to see what's going on – so no pyjamas.

The Jeans Test

The ultimate test! Everyone has an item of clothing that they long to get back into. What's yours? Hang it up somewhere you can see it. When I was losing my baby weight after CoCo, I hung up my favourite Roland Mouret dress where I could see it every day. But the day I finally jumped with joy was when I got back into my skinny jeans, without having to lie down on my bed, breathe in and wiggle them on. When they slip on with ease, you've done it!

Let's be honest: we all want to be healthier and have more energy and live a longer life. But we want to do it wearing the best clothes that we possibly can. It's likely that you will drop one-and-a-half dress sizes per six-week round of your programme. Keep going, keep buying skinnier jeans, and stop when the magic has happened. Clothes are a very accurate indication of results. Don't stop at the jeans you still feel a bit 'blah' in – aim for the ultimate jeans.

Feeling Fabulous

This is the hardest thing to measure but the best feeling there is. You're going to have moments when you feel like the programme isn't working and contemplate turning to the Pity Pot. Keep telling yourself it's a temporary situation and that nothing worth having comes without some effort. Just keep going. Don't stop, no matter what.

You'll know you've reached your goal when you feel fabulous. What's better than having a spring in your step and everyone around you telling you that you look *amazing*? (Your fake friends will tell you that you look gaunt, so be aware of their jealous words and let them blow over you.) You'll glow so brightly they will probably think you are having an affair.

Weigh Yourself ONCE a Fortnight

You're going to weigh yourself **once a fortnight only** – using either body-composition scales or standard bathroom scales. You're going to confine those scales to a cupboard, and don't even think about jumping on them more often. Your body weight goes up and down, even on a radical body-transformation programme, so the only thing you are doing by weighing yourself often is confusing yourself. And if you get a reading you're not happy with, you're going to think the programme isn't working, when it is (because it simply cannot fail to work), and you'll be tempted to jump on the Pity Pot and destroy your motivation. So: **once a fortnight only** and, even then, it's just an indication; you are looking for a trend that's heading downwards.

Start Once

I know I have made this point consistently (there's that word again), but before you start you need to make sure that your mindset is ready. Make your decision to **start once** and just not to stop until you have reached your goal. The programme gathers pace, enthusiasm and speed with every day that you embrace it fully. Remind yourself that this requires 100 per cent commitment for only a matter of weeks. Don't start until you have really committed; but, when you do, remember that you **start once**, stay in the inner circle, learn the dance steps and don't stop until you reach your goal. Take pride in each day you tick off.

Start once and just don't stop

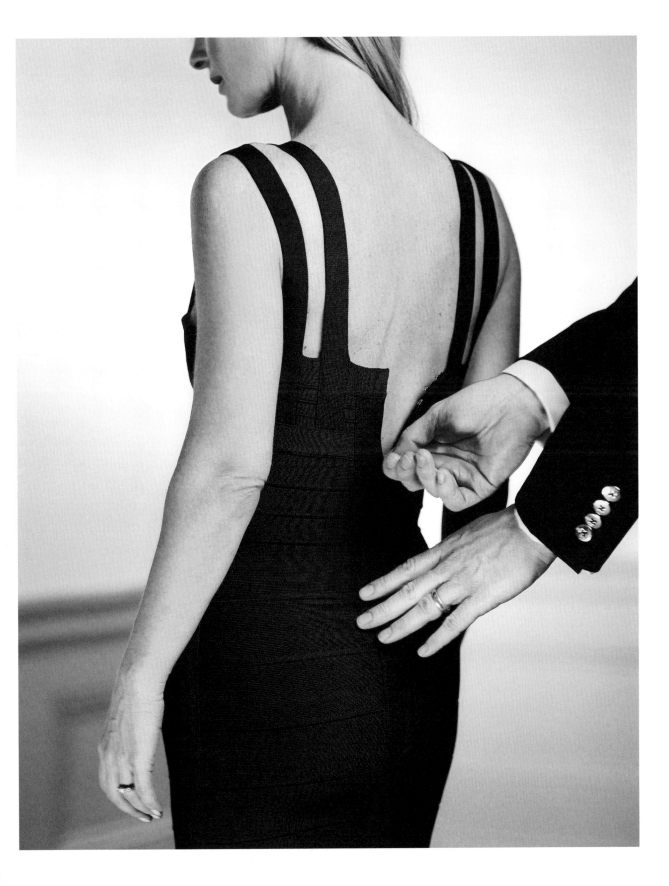

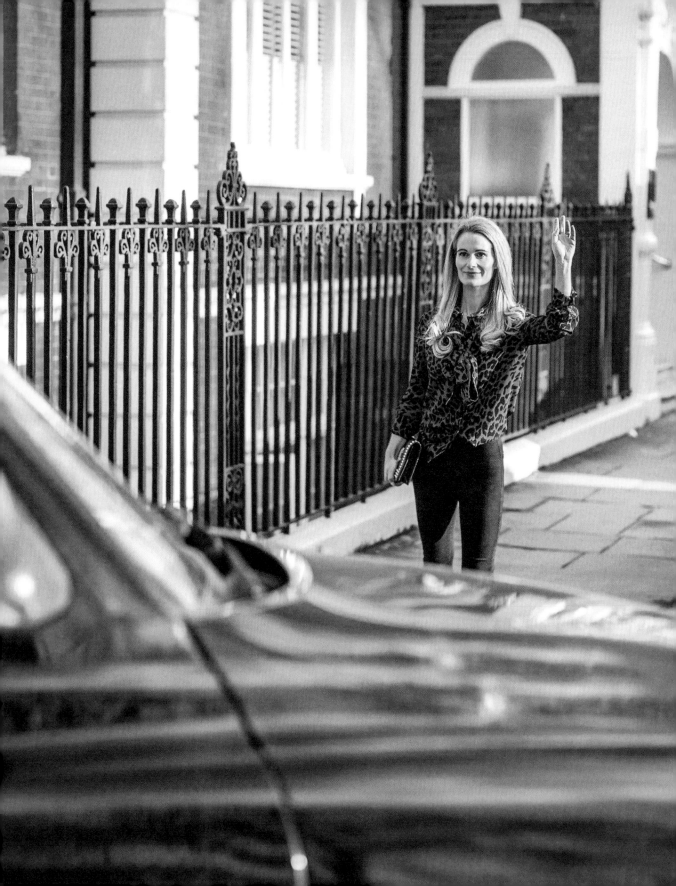

During the Transform Phase

Throughout your programme your job is to stay bang in the middle of the inner circle until you reach your goal. As you progress through Transform there will be times when it feels so easy to stay in this inner circle that you will think you're doing something wrong – you're not; this is a great sign that your programme is fitting you perfectly, both now and for the long term.

'The Four-day Rule'

We are going to get you into this fat-burning inner circle and keep you there for 42 consecutive days – or longer, if you have more weight to lose. There are no days off or 'treat days' on my Method. Here's why.

Depending on the indiscretion, it can take two to three days in the inner circle to get you back into the fat-burning zone. So every time you take yourself out of the inner circle, you turn the fat-burning tap off, the clock resets and it takes two to three days to get things started again. So if you take one day fully 'OFF' the programme and out of the inner circle, it will take three days of being 'ON' the programme to get the fat-burning tap dripping again. So you lose four days in total.

If you do this five times throughout a six-week programme, you essentially lose 20 days of a 42-day programme and will gain less than 50 per cent of the optimum result.

Think of that fat-burning tap – you want it to drip steadily, every day for six weeks, rather than be turned on and off the whole time, which will reduce your results by half.

So when you have more challenging moments in the Transform Phase, try to think of the dance: visualize the inner circle and stay focused that your one job is to remain inside it. Try not to step outside it, and don't let anyone push you out. Be stubborn, be determined, be proud and really focus on staying in.

Cheats & Treats

If you do pop out of the inner circle (a glass of wine, a couple of biscuits or a day or two of missed exercise), do not panic. It is not the end of the world. Simply jump straight back into the inner circle, because your aim is to spend as much time as possible here.

The more time you spend in the inner circle and the less time in the outer circle, the sooner you will 'get the habit' and the more fabulous your results will be. The easiest route is the most direct route, and the most direct route is totally worth it, once your results really kick in.

Don't Stop Before the Magic Happens

Before you make the switch from Transform to Lifestyle, be sure that you've reached your ultimate goal. Make sure you're standing in the body that you visualized before your move into the Lifestyle Plan. **Remember: maintaining a size-8 body is no more challenging than maintaining a size-14 one – it just takes a little longer to get there.** Your body is maintaining its current fat levels, dropping body fat or gaining fat, regardless of what size you are. So don't for one moment think that you cannot aim for a smaller dress size and worry that you'll find it harder to sustain a leaner body. It won't make a blind bit of difference.

I personally don't buy into the idea that you have to be fatter when you're 60 than you were at 30. It makes no sense to me. The idea that you have to choose between your face and your body is nonsense. This was the case in the 1980s, when dieting was all about non-fat and high-carbohydrate foods – which have the most detrimental effect on skin, instigated by the lack of good oils that maintain beauty, and an excess of sugars that accelerate skin ageing in a dramatic way.

So put this myth aside. I've seen hundreds of clients in their fifties, sixties and seventies regain a body that surpasses the figure they had in their thirties, and not once have I looked at their faces and thought they've looked 'drawn'. As long as you're looking after your skin by wearing SPF, using anti-ageing serums and eating a diet rich in antioxidants, protein and omega oils, you're going to look fabulous. So don't use your face as a reason not to ditch another dress size. I'll say it again: get the body that thrills you. Make sure you are not standing in your own way.

Please, please don't get off the train one stop too early. Aim for your best-ever body – it's what I really want for you, and there's no reason why you can't have it. The only thing that might prevent you reaching the very best version of yourself is the limitation in your own mind – so believe that you can take your body one step further, if that's what you'd love. Our bodies are simply a creation of what we put into them and how we move them, so you are in control of your figure and how you feel.

How Do I Know I'm Ready to Switch to the Louise Parker Lifestyle?

Turn now to your 'Before' and 'After' photographs (see page 204) and look at them with a compassionate, logical and realistic eye. If you're overcritical and body-dysmorphic, then you need to ask a friend (the one who would tell you if you'd got spinach in your teeth) to be totally honest with you.

Think back to your visualization. It was hopefully the very best aesthetic version of you – so your body in the best physical shape that it can be – and not a 5½ft 22-year-old if you're 45 and nudging 5ft. It's you, with all the tone that you desire with your body-fat levels just where you wanted them to be.

Only you can decide when you've reached a body-fat level that pleases you and suits your frame. Once we ease you into the Lifestyle Plan, your fat-burning tap will slowly turn off. As you make the transition, you need to be at the point where your body-fat levels are where you want them to be. So, are you as lean as you'd like to be? Is there more fat on your body that you'd like to lose?

You may find that you still have a little pocket of fat somewhere that isn't in perfect balance with the rest of your body. This is common: 95 per cent of women that I see in my clinic in their underwear have a stubborn fat-pocket somewhere – so remember to focus on the best version of yourself, not on perfection. Perfection does not exist. Even models don't look like models – all the little bumps and pockets of imperfection are airbrushed away with fury.

You cannot 'spot-fat reduce'. Targeting a stubborn little pocket of fat through diet, lifestyle and exercise is physically impossible. Your body will reduce body fat all over when you are losing fat, and you can't direct where it will let go of fat. If, for example, you've a little bump on the outer thigh, doing outer-thigh exercises will help to tone the muscle beneath the fat, but they won't burn the fat on top of it.

Given that no one can spot-fat reduce and we wouldn't want to make you underweight to target this pocket, you've got two options. You can either look towards a non-invasive cosmetic treatment such as cool-sculpting (which is expensive but effective for small stubborn pockets of fat, but not an overall weight-loss solution) or embrace the fact that you've worked your socks off to get the best body you can – and it's utterly fabulous.

This is important: you need to look at your body with a logical eye and acknowledge what is body fat that can be burned by staying on Transform, what is a stubborn fat-pocket (whilst the rest of you is as lean as you'd like it to be) and what can be improved by further sculpting your figure through a commitment to the ongoing workouts, whilst not losing any more body fat.

It might be that you're as lean as you'd like to be all over, with a teeny pocket of fat on your thighs, but you'd like further definition in your legs, stomach and arms. If you want to sculpt your body further, but recognize that it's time to turn off the fat-burning tap, then switch to Lifestyle – and continue with your workouts.

Your body will continue to evolve, sculpting a more beautiful physique, the longer you live the Lifestyle Plan. By continually innovating and changing up the workout routines, your muscles are going to tighten and keep on improving. So the physical shape and lines of your body will continue to improve, whilst your body-fat levels stabilize.

I want you to have the best body ever – and there is no reason why you can't have it

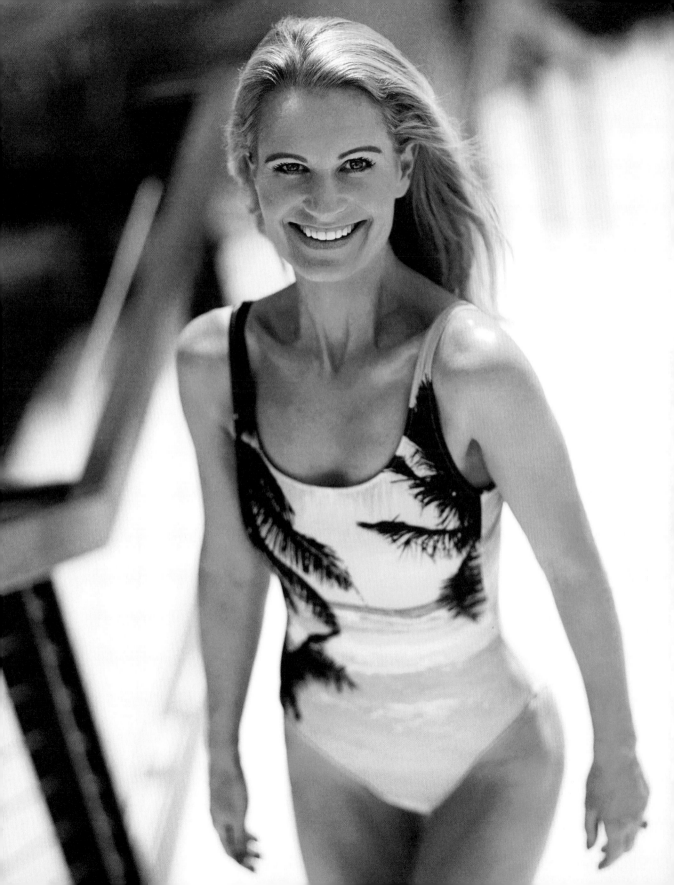

THE LOUISE
PARKER
LIFESTYLE

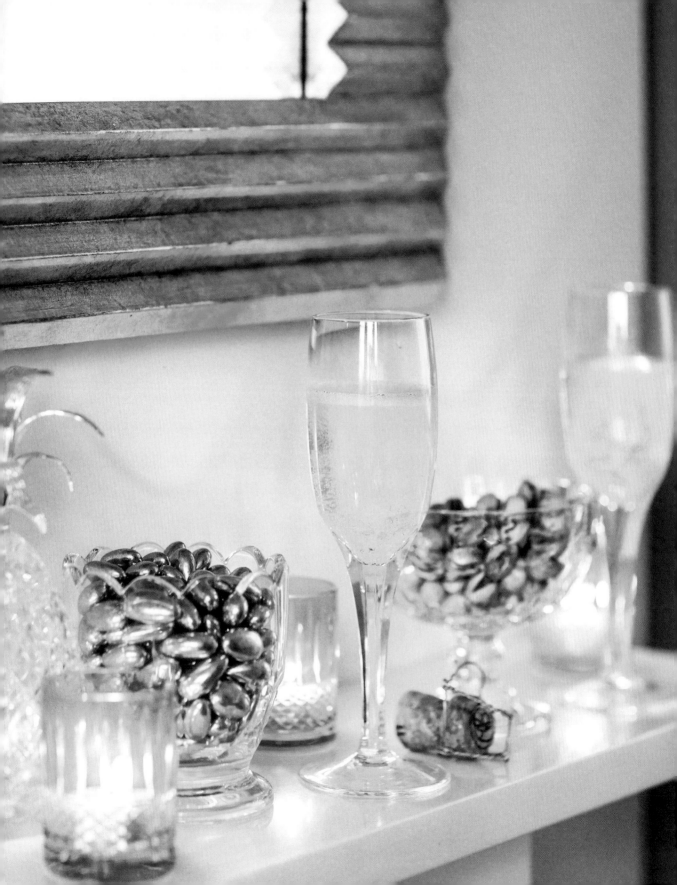

Your New Normal

Everything you learn in the Transform Phase will form the foundation of your New Normal. Whilst you've been shrinking and sculpting your body, you've been creating habits that will last a lifetime. The beautiful meals and the habit of exercise will now form part of your life – and just be what you do now. You'll continue with a positive mindset and lifestyle habits and will really take pleasure in looking after yourself.

You'll find your own balance of what works for you, to perfectly maintain your results in the most effortless way, whilst still enjoying the celebratory foods and drinks that are 'worth it' to you. You'll continue to innovate through workouts that progress, and will keep fine-tuning good habits so that you live your best life in your best body.

The Lifestyle Plan is about freedom from trend dieting and learning the art of maintaining a lean body in the most intelligent, effortless and lovable way. It's about living the forever habits of balance and brilliance – in mindset, lifestyle *and* body.

★ Maintain a positive mindset and continually innovate your lifestyle.

★ Eat to the Louise Parker Method Food Plan 80 per cent of the time.

★ Enjoy celebratory food and drinks 20 per cent of the time absolutely guilt-free.

★ Continue with a minimum of 10,000 steps per day.

★ Work out daily.

★ Continue your Digital Detox after 9pm every night.

★ Innovate your workouts every six weeks.

★ Sleep for seven hours a night.

★ Deal with all your worries head-on, with a 'Do it Now' attitude.

★ Make time for simple pleasures every single day.

★ Keep positive, inspiring company and help others to Transform.

★ Take 20 minutes a day to 'brain-nap'.

I love the way my programmes take you to your goal with a body that just thrills you and a new lifestyle that has *simultaneously* fallen into place. Each and every habit that you've practised throughout Transform you will continue with: it's simply what you do now. Nothing comes to a grinding halt and there's no going back to your past habits, which – when you think about them now – probably feel as if they were part of someone else.

You won't *want* to go back, because you will be feeling the best version of yourself – physically strong and lean, mentally sharp and positive, and living a life that's ordered, calm and continues to challenge you in a good way. You are simply going to pop in all the celebratory foods and drinks that make your life an absolute pleasure – but only when they are fabulous and really 'worth it'. I'll show you how to do this, and it'll be much easier than you think.

My Lifestyle Plan gives you the freedom from trend dieting forever

How to Transition Between Transform & Lifestyle/The Dance

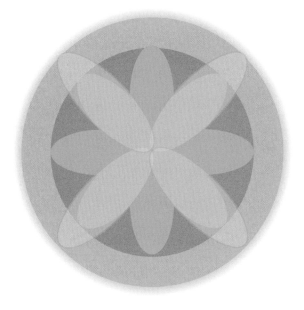

The difference between Transform and Lifestyle is simply spending 80 per cent in the inner circle, rather than the 100 per cent you have been doing throughout Transform.

Now, I use these percentages loosely, and you are not about to start doing complicated mathematics, but to rely on common sense. You want a perfect balance that keeps you as lean as you love to be. It will take you two or three weeks to work out how much time you can spend in the outer circle and to stabilize your body-fat levels.

Everybody is different, and I want you to transition slowly as you find your balance. This is how you do it:

Establish Your Repertoire

I think everyone needs about 10 or 20 favourites that form the basic repertoire of what they eat on a day-to-day basis. I want you to continually evolve your repertoire, trying new things, so that you don't get stuck in a rut of eating the same four things for lunch every week. But it's important to know what your favourites are, so that they form the basis of your habits – and you can continually tweak them.

Step back and decide what your ongoing eating habits are going to be, so that you can shop, prepare and enjoy without having to think about it too much. For example, you may have swapped sugar-laden Special K for my Bircher breakfasts, which come in endless varieties. Birchers would then become part of your repertoire.

Make a list of all the recipes you have learned and loved throughout your Transform programme – including breakfast, snacks, lunches and evening meals. You'll keep evolving your favourites and innovating your meals with delicious variety.

Now Define Your 'Worth Its'

As you go through Transform, situations will arise that challenge you – and, through these situations, you will soon realize what celebratory meals and drinks you truly miss. You need to recognize what foods and drinks belonging in the middle and outer circles are 'worth it' to you – and which ones you honestly want to reintroduce into your life. Clients often say to me in the honeymoon period of finishing a transformation, 'Oh, I could eat like this for ever – I don't miss a thing' and it always raises a red flag for me.

Living in the real world means that you'll want to cuddle up in front of the fire with a glass of wine and a bowl of pretzels; order whatever makes your heart sing when you're in your favourite restaurant; and enjoy the roast potatoes on a Sunday. And so you should: my Method is not about deprivation. Define what you have really missed – what the 'worth its' are to you – and ink them. I'm looking for a list of foods that are about celebration, no matter how simple they are, and not a list of all your favourite chocolate bars. Be discerning. You've worked hard to get your new body, and now you have to decide what foods are worthy of you.

If you're a frequent business traveller, I highly recommend that you nail 'eating beautifully' whilst travelling as part of your programme. It *can* be done; it just takes a little more planning and adaptation. When you crack it, you'll see that it's so much more 'worth it' having your celebrations with loved ones and family than eating crisps at 30,000ft.

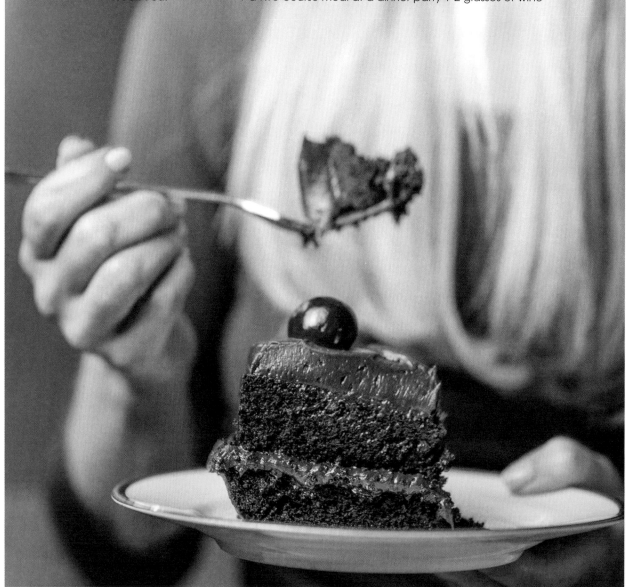

Now Ease into Your 'Worth Its'

Perhaps you have a list of ten 'worth its'. They might be events, rather than a specific meal, which is fine. You want to slowly introduce your celebrations (not 'treats' or 'cheats') so that you can see how your body adjusts. You'll introduce a couple each week, and you'll know you've hit the right balance when you've introduced all your celebrations and your body stabilizes. Here is an example of how I ease back into my 'New Normal' after a post-natal transformation, taking a month to get there:

★ **Week One**   2 glasses of wine on a Friday night

★ **Week Two**   + a Sunday roast with all the trimmings

★ **Week Three**   + 2 pancakes and maple syrup on a Saturday morning

★ **Week Four**   + a two-course meal at a dinner party + 2 glasses of wine

This is a good indication of what I can get away with on a weekly basis, but of course it's not set in stone – I go by what my weekly events are. And the longer I've lived this way, the easier it has become to be discerning and choose wisely.

It's not something I agonize over. I simply eat whatever a social situation steers me towards and what my body craves. You will often find that in a restaurant you actually want to eat according to the Method, because you just get used to eating in a cleaner, lighter way. Often I look forward to a ribeye steak and chips, then end up leaving half the chips and wishing there was a larger salad.

The Lowdown on Socializing

Many a time I've sat across the table from someone and they've said, 'God, you're so lucky – if I ate that, I'd be the size of a house.' And, you know, I probably said that many a time too, before I learned what I know now. What they don't see is that 80 per cent of the time I'm living my Method, so I can afford to tuck into a crème brûlée and a glass of Sancerre without my weight fluctuating.

Whether you can get away with 20 or 30 per cent of your time in celebration depends on how active you are. If your regular workouts are sporadic for a few weeks, you'll have to rein it in a bit. When you're training consistently, you'll probably get away with 30 per cent.

I'm not going to tell you exactly how many celebrations you can indulge in, or make a list of what 20 or 30 per cent looks like. You have to work it out for yourself and trust your instinct on this – it's sharper than you think. Soon you'll really enjoy being able to casually calibrate what works for your own body. Your body will tell you far better than I can, so listen to it.

At the start of every week see what you have coming up – how many meals out, soirées and other events. If you're out every night, you will have to balance it by eating clean and lean during the day and just keep your wits about you each evening to moderate what you eat and drink. If you're out three times, you'll probably get away with letting your hair down a little on each of those evenings. It takes a bit of time to learn what your individual body responds well to, and you should do this slowly, thoughtfully and carefully – until it becomes second nature.

Be aware of how much alcohol you are drinking, if that's your thing. Booze will tempt you into the outer circle, before you know it. It's packed full of sugar, stimulates your appetite and, most of all, mentally weakens you so that you don't even care. It's a good idea to have a 'two-glass rule', so that your habit when you're socializing is simply to stick to two glasses of your favourite tipple and thoroughly enjoy it. I can't promise I do this every night out – but as a general rule it works.

Of course there are going to be events when you let your hair down – but we're talking here about your regular routine. And if you can make this one of your new habits, you'll avoid regularly overindulging and all the collateral damage of hangovers, let alone all the things you shouldn't have said.

Let Go of 'Cheat Meals'

I want you to totally erase terms such as 'cheat meals', 'treats', 'sins' or anything that suggests that something you eat is 'naughty' in any way. With my Method you live in balance, with clean, lean meals and richer, more extravagant meals and moments – and none of these are forbidden. I really, really mean this and it can make or break whether you 'get' my method of permanent weight loss or remain a constant dieter. You won't make 'organically overweight' cake unless you want to; you can simply eat normal cake.

You have to let go of thinking like this, as it drives a negative mindset, which only gets you down and leads towards remorse and self-sabotage. I want you to eat an almond croissant without thinking of it as 'naughty'. **An almond croissant is just that, and a totally normal part of eating. I cringe now when I hear anyone say that they 'cheated' – it's simply a turn in the dance. You will learn to embrace a weekend in Paris, eating what your heart desires, in a beautiful way that feels extravagant and luxurious, and not a case of remorseful overindulgence.**

Continue to Innovate Your Lifestyle

You're going to continue to innovate your Lifestyle Plan so that you evolve, stay highly motivated and inspired, and embrace your new lifestyle with passion. I tend to think in terms of school term-times, and each half-term I mix up my routine a bit. However you divide your year, make marks in your diary to prompt you to review things – the change of the seasons is a great reminder. You have to take time and give some thought to refreshing your plan – not in a totally obsessive way, but just to keep it feeling inventive and fresh. If you don't, the risk is that your motivation will plateau and dwindle, followed by your results. So really take this on board.

Keep Evolving Your Repertoire of Favourite Meals

Now that you understand the principles of my Method, you will be able to devise many of your own recipes and family favourites. The recipe options that nod towards the Method are almost endless, and those included in this book are just the start. The possibilities are endless.

It's a good habit to sit down once a month and jot down a list of all your favourite recipes – making sure each month that, out of the list of 10 or 20 for each meal, at least a third of them are new. Keep evolving it and keep it interesting. You'll naturally want to eat more seasonally anyway and go with what your body craves. My Method is not about eating the same meals every day – keep inventing, and do it with passion. Experiment, have fun and don't be afraid to make mistakes.

Keep Evolving Your Workouts

By continually innovating and changing the workout routines, your body is going to continually evolve. You'll become stronger, more flexible and sculpted as your body-fat levels stabilize. There's always something to be worked on: see yourself as an ongoing project. I'm always working towards something – whether it's flexibility, pushing myself to try something that's totally out of my comfort zone, or focusing in on a part of my body that's out of balance and needs correcting, for postural or couture reasons.

As you improve your muscle tone over the coming months, your basal metabolic rate will also get a boost, which means that you have the option of adding in even more recipes in celebration. Evolving your workout routine is just as much about keeping your mind engaged as your muscles. Your body improves with 'muscle confusion' – so challenge your body with new exercises, angles and activities. If you fail to evolve your routine, your body will cease to evolve. But, more importantly, if you follow the same routine every week for months, you'll die of boredom and start slacking off your habits.

It's for this reason that I mix up my routine every half-term – working also with the seasons and with what I have coming up in my diary. Before Christmas or the summer holidays I'll probably increase my training by 30 per cent to ensure that I'm in the best shape possible. But it's very motivating to have a goal to push you out of your comfort zone, force you to be accountable to yourself and inject some renewed passion into your regime. Keep your body *and* mind stimulated – I think it's healthy to up your ambitions every now and again.

Continue to evolve your workouts; it will keep your mind and muscles stimulated

Healthy Holiday Habits

Holidays on the Louise Parker Method are no different from being on the Lifestyle Plan. Because the lifestyle is my habit, I habitually live by my 80/20-ish rule on holiday, too. I don't really think about it. I prefer to come home feeling refreshed and not sluggish from overconsumption. But that's not to say that I don't have an extremely good time – I do.

On holiday, for example, without really thinking about it, I eat to my Method at breakfast and lunch and venture out to the outer circle in the evening, for a couple of glasses of wine or a clam risotto, if it's 'worth it'. If the croissants are amazing, I'll have a croissant at breakfast, then eat in the inner circle for the rest of the day – perhaps popping into the outer circle for a cocktail or two later on. I move every single day. I probably do more exercise just playing with the girls and make time for long walks on the beach.

I might have a couple of evenings outside the circle: a lavish meal, a few cocktails and a coconut ice-cream, which is one of my 'worth its'. If something doesn't properly seduce me, then I don't bother eating it. In the end it all balances out, and I never put on a pound on holiday. In the old days I'd write off the whole two weeks, spend most of it outside the circle and come home 7lb the worse for wear – and get back on the diet treadmill.

I go without nothing that I truly crave on holiday, or in life in general. If I want it, I have it – and dance straight back into the inner circle. It's become such a habit that I don't even need to think about it. Once you've practised it on your first holiday, you'll be amazed how easy you find it and how thrilled that you're flying home feeling your absolute best.

The Three-day Rule

Life, thankfully, is full of celebration. You're going to continue to love all the indulgences of Christmas, New Year, your birthday in Paris and your best friend's wedding weekend. You are human, and you're going to have days when you let rip. Don't overthink it or make it a big deal. You can take it too seriously, which will make you stumble on your dance moves. Just remember that Christmas, your birthday in Paris, your anniversary weekend means three days – and not three weeks – written off. It's absolutely okay to spend a handful of days in the middle and outer circles. Just live by the three-day rule: don't stay there longer than three days. On Day Four you head straight back to the inner circle.

The same applies to your workouts. You will, of course, have days when for one reason or another you simply cannot get your head around a workout. I really want you to get into the habit of doing a little something every day, but even I have times when I simply can't muster the motivation. We're not aiming for perfection. Simply apply the same three-day rule: if you've sat on your backside for three days, on the fourth day – no matter what – you get up and do something; even if it's just 20 minutes, it will be enough to get you going again. This is a really important rule that will affect your backside for ever.

Monitoring Your Results

Just as you did throughout your programme, I want you to continue to monitor your results. Once you have reached your goal, continue to follow the same monitoring routine. After six months of consolidating, monthly results will be enough. It's important to track your progress throughout your transformation and, as you ease into Lifestyle, so you should continue to calibrate your balance, although I don't want you to become obsessive.

Once you're in the body you love, buy yourself some skinny jeans. Make sure they're tight. Fitting into your skinny jeans – and by that I mean pulling them on in 30 seconds, not a lying-down operation that takes five minutes – is the simplest, and probably most accurate, way of monitoring your results long-term. The longer you live in your best body, the easier it becomes. You'll just know when it's time to up it to 90 per cent for a few weeks or inject more into your workouts.

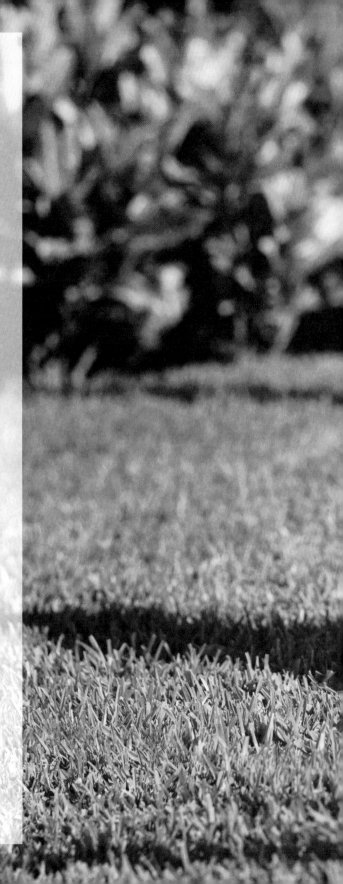

Afterword

I hope that you find in the Louise Parker Method the strength, freedom and joy that I have, and that it becomes your New Normal too.

What I wish for you is that you find the same liberation from dieting as I have, and replace self-sabotage and sacrifice with strength and permanent success. I'm confident that the Method will become a part of you, as it has of me. Remember: it's not a temporary programme, but simply how you now choose to live.

Living my Method and passing it on has undoubtedly made me a better version of myself – far beyond the physical aspect. I have the energy, enthusiasm and mindset to take the most challenging days in my stride.

I've learned so much from thousands of inspiring clients over 20 years – each and every one enduring their own little struggles. Don't think you're the only one who finds it tricky from time to time. You can do this. I know you can.

Never give up. Think of it like breathing: if you stop, then the motivation and magic will dwindle. Keep continuing to take in shallow breaths, when you have days that test you – the tiniest effort will be enough to sustain you, until you have a day when you can breathe deeply again.

Such is the ebb and flow of life; you are not aiming for perfection, for it does not exist. To aim for perfection is to tell yourself that you're not capable of change.

Keep recalling what I said about 'The Dance' and 'Consistency, Not Severity' and that it must never feel like displeasure. Let go, once and for all, of the 'all-or-nothing' mindset that has held you back for years, and instead head directly to your goal as swiftly as you can, and learn to enjoy the dance. You must find the pleasure in it. It's there – you simply have to open yourself up to it.

Treat yourself as you would your child or your friend: mother yourself, when you feel you need it. It's not a race – it's just a dance. And if you remember to keep moving towards your goal, no matter what, you will reach the happiest, most vibrant version of your already brilliant self.

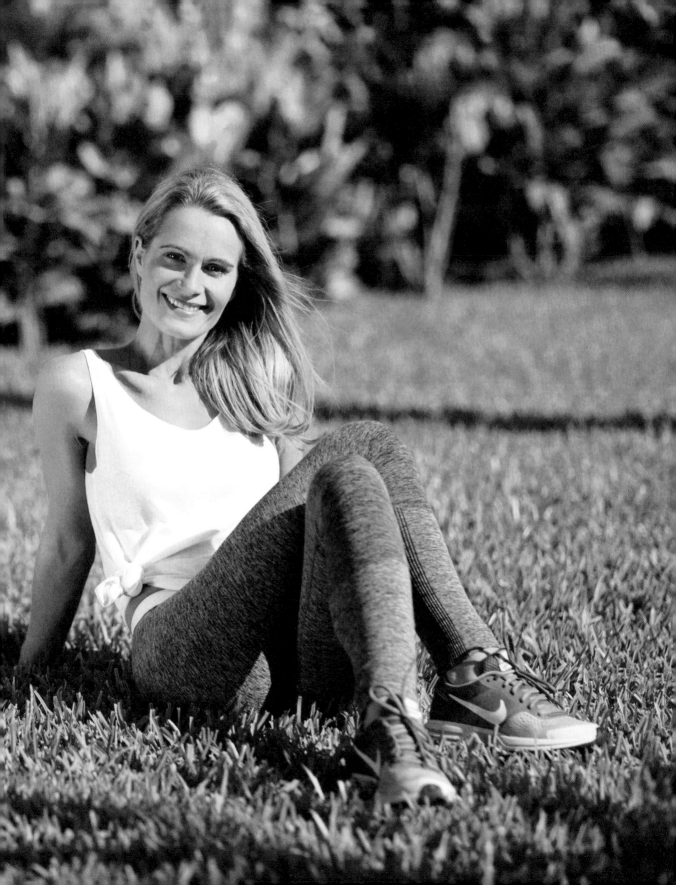

INDEX

ACKNOWLEDGEMENTS

My deepest gratitude goes to my husband Paul. I'm forever grateful that you quit your 'proper job' in the City, dedicating yourself from day one to our baby family business. You are the most loving, wonderful and bright person I know. I could not do it without you and it is testament to our marriage that we live, love and laugh so happily with our lives so intertwined. Thank you for being a feminist and a devoted husband and father. I love you more each week.

To my phenomenal daughters Sophie, Emily and Chloe. You've carried me to the finish line with your love, optimism and unwavering encouragement through the trials and tribulations of what has, at times, felt like birthing my fourth child. Your daily motivation and pride in 'mummy's work' has softened the pain of my distance from you these last few months. May you lean in to every opportunity and challenge that comes your way.

I give continual gratitude to my loving family. My parents, John Maynard FRCS and Josephine Maynard, have given me every opportunity one could wish for alongside constant encouragement and unfaltering love through thick and thin. Thank you for giving me the freedom to make mistakes and learn my lessons. I am inspired by your professionalism, humility (yet to rub off), values (work in progress) and how very hard you worked for us, to provide us with the best that life can offer – often at great cost to yourselves. I am trying to pass this on.

I'm beyond grateful to our Nonna and Pa and Nick and Angela. You couldn't wish for a better family in law and we owe so much to you for your constant support, love and laughter. You've jumped to the rescue more times than I can recall and I cherish you more than I remember to say. You are the definition of love and I thank you for providing me with the best father and husband.

My brothers, Johnny and Rees, will always be my grounding force and I love both them and their families with all that I am. I know you would move mountains for me or tell me how to do it myself. You know when to lift me up or take me down a peg or three, and I couldn't be without you. I'm blessed to now have sisters I adore and an army of nieces and nephews who make my heart sing.

My dearest friends, most of whom are scattered around the globe, have been loving, loyal and fabulous and have patiently understood my flakiness these last few months. Thank you for doing so with such grace. I won't list you by name, but you know who you are. I love each and every one of you like a sister.

Many phenomenal women have mentored and inspired me throughout my career and I thank them all wholeheartedly. My dear friends Sian Davies, Dr. Dambisa Moyo, Sandi Toksvig OBE, Leslie Zabala, Baroness Ann Jenkin, Lady Sarah Stacey, Gavanndra Hodge, and more recently Nicky Kinnaird MBE. You all inspire me to keep going and kick arse. I thank too, Jane Fonda, for it is your arse that inspired me in this direction years ago at boarding school when I set up my little fitness club, after *Neighbours* each day.

My work family at Louise Parker really are just that. I thank you all equally for your passion and commitment, and for making coming to work such a pleasure. I thank the outstanding personal trainers on my team who set their alarms so early and work their socks off with dedication and professionalism every single day.

Lauren has done such a good job of recruiting the best of the best that I don't have space to thank the army of you. You all make me proud. Special thanks to Christle Coxton (soon to be Dr), Alejandra McCall RDA, Amelie Gonguet, Catherine Fallon, Tara Jones, Lauren Rand and Emma Holyoake for holding the fort so fabulously in my absence. We are the sum of all our parts and I thank each and every one of you to the moon and back.

I thank my agent – the best in the business – Heather Holden Brown for nudging me all these years to write this book and actually making it happen. I've felt in the hands of a loving friend and matron throughout and without you, this book would never have been written. I'm indebted to you.

An enormous thanks to my publisher, Octopus, at Hachette, who were cheerleaders of this book from the moment we met. My brilliant commissioning editor, Eleanor Maxfield, was Chief Cheerleader. She immediately 'got' our method from our first meeting and ensured that my somewhat perfectionist demands were always listened to patiently yet with sensible judgement. Yasia Williams deserves a bloody medal for art directing and somehow getting this beautiful book to print on time, despite my somewhat demanding personality. You are both incredibly talented, patient and a huge pleasure to work with. I'm very grateful to the whole team at Octopus who were behind the scenes night and day helping us give birth. Leanne Bryan, Caroline Alberti, Karen Baker, Frances Teehan, Marianne Laidlaw, Stuart Lemon and the bearded Kevin Hawkins – you have all been beyond fabulous.

Huge gratitude to the beautiful Natalie Thompson for your incredible culinary artistry and positivity, and for making all my simple recipes look do-able yet gorgeous. Thanks also to the talented Louise Hagger for capturing them so beautifully and calmly in her dungarees; your photos are a delight, as are you. A heartfelt hug to Tabitha Hawkins for your outstanding styling and for pushing my grey boundaries to perfection. I thank photographer Rodrigo del Rio Lozano in Mexico for his amazing work – you and Eileen were a great pleasure to be with.

Shooting our fitness and family pictures in London was damn hard work in freezing conditions, and yet Chris Terry managed to capture our life so beautifully, putting us all at ease and keeping us laughing throughout the day. I loved working with you. Thank you to the hair and make up genius Maria Comparetto who is usually tending to models, not little mums like me.

People often ask 'How do you juggle it all? The honest answer is, I don't. Winnie Dopale and Emma Holyoake keep my home and work life so beautifully synched that I just about manage to squeeze it all in. I love you and thank you for going way beyond the call of duty for all these years. You are my rocks.

Last, but most importantly, I thank each and every client of Louise Parker who has completed a programme with us. Many of you have become very dear friends to Paul, the children and I. You provide us all with the enthusiasm to work harder each day and you show us that anything is possible.

Love to all of you. It's been bloody hard work, but an absolute joy.

An Hachette UK Company
www.hachette.co.uk

First published in Great Britain in 2016 by Mitchell Beazley,
a division of Octopus Publishing Group Ltd, Carmelite
House, 50 Victoria Embankment, London EC4Y 0DZ
www.octopusbooks.co.uk
www.octopusbooksusa.com

Design & layout copyright © Octopus Publishing
Group Ltd 2016
Text copyright © Louise Parker Limited 2016
Food photography copyright © Louise Hagger 2016
Lifestyle photography, plus the image on page 17,
copyright © Chris Terry 2016
Photography on pages 6, 13, 29, 152–3, 159, 209 and
218–19 copyright © Louise Parker Limited 2016

Distributed in the US by Hachette Book Group,
1290 Avenue of the Americas, 4th and 5th Floors,
New York, NY 10020

Distributed in Canada by Canadian Manda Group,
664 Annette St, Toronto, Ontario, Canada M6S 2C8

All rights reserved. No part of this work may be reproduced
or utilized in any form or by any means, electronic or
mechanical, including photocopying, recording or by any
information storage and retrieval system, without the
prior written permission of the publisher.

Louise Parker asserts the moral right to be identified as
the author of this work.

ISBN 978-1-78472-175-6

A CIP catalogue record for this book is available from
the British Library.

Printed and bound in China.

10 9 8 7 6 5 4 3

All reasonable care has been taken in the preparation of
this book, but the information it contains is not meant to
take the place of medical care under the direct supervision
of a doctor. Before making any changes in your health and
fitness regime, always consult a doctor. Any application of
the ideas and information contained in this book is at the
reader's sole discretion and risk. Neither the author nor the
publisher will be responsible for any injury, loss, damages,
actions, proceedings, claims, demands, expenses and costs
(including legal costs or expenses) incurred in any way
arising out of following the exercises in this book.

Publisher's Acknowledgements

Commissioning Editor Eleanor Maxfield
Art Director Yasia Williams-Leedham
Designers Yasia Williams-Leedham and Geoff Fennell
Senior Editor Leanne Bryan
Copy Editor Mandy Greenfield
Photographers Louise Hagger and Chris Terry
Illustrator Soleil Ignacio
Food Stylist Natalie Thompson
Prop Stylist Tabitha Hawkins
Hair & Make–up Maria Comparetto
Head Stylist Nicole Leech
Assistant Stylist Gina Stewart
Production Controller Allison Gonsalves

The publisher would like to thank the following for
their contributions to this book:

Laain www.laain.co.uk
Rainbow Wave www.rainbowwave.com
Pia Auld www.piahallstrom.com
Fabric PR www.fabricpr.com

Picture Credits

Cover photography Front: far left & spine, Rodrigo del
Rio Lozano; centre left above & below, Louise Hagger;
centre right above, Louise Hagger; centre right below,
Chris Terry; far right, Rodrigo del Rio Lozano. Back: far
left & centre left, Chris Terry; centre right above & below,
Louise Hagger; far right, Rodrigo del Rio Lozano.

All food photography Louise Hagger, except for page
17, Chris Terry; **All lifestyle photography** Chris Terry,
except for pages 6, 13, 29, 152–3, 159, 209 and 218–19,
Rodrigo del Rio Lozano.